T0274763

Medicinal Plants of the Pacific Northwest

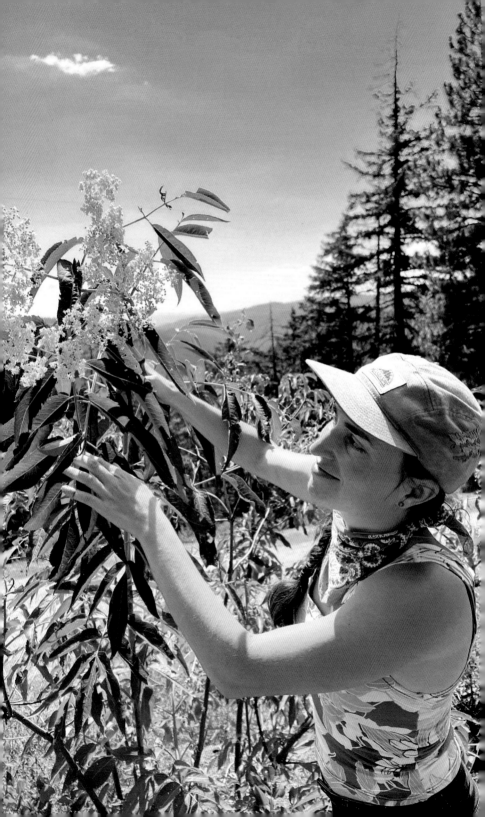

Medicinal Plants of the Pacific Northwest

A Visual Guide to Harvesting and Healing with 35 Common Species

Natalie Hammerquist

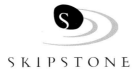

SKIPSTONE

Published by Skipstone, an imprint of Mountaineers Books—an independent, nonprofit publisher.
Skipstone and its colophon are registered trademarks of The Mountaineers organization.

Printed in China

27 26 25 24   1 2 3 4 5

Design: Melissa McFeeters
Cover photographs, clockwise from top left: *Oregon grape berries*; *Stream violet* (Ben Legler); *Hawthorn flower*; *Elderflower syrup*; *Yarrow flowers*; *Cramp bark flowers*; *Cedar smoke stick*; *Gumweed flower*; *California poppy* (Wren Morrow); *Western redcedar leaf*
Photographs: page 8, *Mullein growing among ponderosa pines*; page 259, *An old-growth ponderosa pine tree growing near Roslyn, Washington* (Lukas Speckhardt); page 274, *Narrowleaf plantain*; page 268, *Delphinium menziesii* photos courtesy of iNaturalist; page 285, Author photo by Wren Morrow
All photographs by the author unless otherwise noted.

Disclaimer: Please use common sense. This book is not intended as a substitute for professional instruction. Harvesting, using, and/or eating any wild plant is inherently risky, and it is incumbent upon any user of this guide to assess their own skills and experience and to be aware of any plant-based allergies or similar personal risks. Likewise, readers should assume responsibility for their own actions, including awareness of changing or unfavorable foraging conditions. The author has made every effort to ensure the accuracy of the information in this book; however, herbal and medicinal plant research and knowledge are always evolving. The publisher and author are expressly not responsible for any adverse consequences resulting directly or indirectly from information contained in this book.

Library of Congress Cataloging-in-Publication Data is on file at https://lccn.loc.gov/2023041986. The LC ebook record is available at https://lccn.loc.gov/2023041987.

Printed on FSC-certified materials

ISBN (paperback): 978-1-68051-697-5
ISBN (ebook): 978-1-68051-698-2

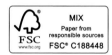

Skipstone books may be purchased for corporate, educational, or other promotional sales, and our authors are available for a wide range of events. For information on special discounts or booking an author, contact our customer service at 800.553.4453 or mbooks@mountaineersbooks.org.

Skipstone
1001 SW Klickitat Way
Suite 201
Seattle, Washington 98134
206.223.6303
www.skipstonebooks.org
www.mountaineersbooks.org

L I V E   L I F E .   M A K E   R I P P L E S .

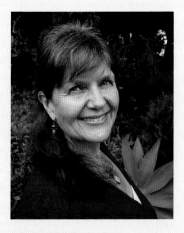

In Memory of Cascade Anderson Geller

Cascade was my first plant-medicine teacher. I met her when I attended a class she taught at an herb fair when I was a senior in college, and I was rapt by the straightforward approach she took to healing with plants. That class had such an impact, I ended up driving all the way to Portland from Olympia one weekend a month to study with her.

She taught in stories, and boy, did she have stories to tell. She told of her grandfather treating local dogs for mange in Appalachia, where she grew up; the home-keeping habits of women in rural villages in Ecuador; finding Oregon grape while trekking in Nepal; finding wild horehound while visiting a Roman bath in Italy; putting aloe on her friend who had been stung by a Portuguese man-of-war in the Mediterranean; and picking lavender in rural France. The stories she told always had a piece of wisdom in them, and I find myself retelling them to my own students in the way that herbalists have always done.

Cascade instilled in me the importance of integrity and activism in the practice of herbalism. She was a fierce advocate for plants, people, and place.

I am able to put this book into the world because of Cascade and all my teachers, and all their teachers, and all their teachers' teachers. Plant-medicine knowledge has always been carried in the hands of the people, weathering many storms against it. Please take this knowledge, experience it, make it your own, and pass it along. Please speak for the plants, like Cascade did. May the hands that carry this knowledge be strong so that it may never be lost.

Contents

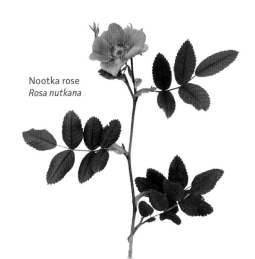

Nootka rose
Rosa nutkana

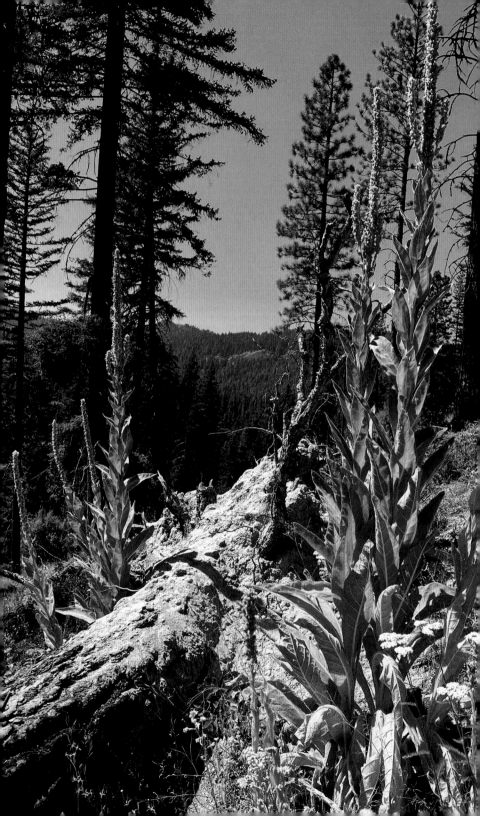

Author's Note

When I was growing up, my father, thoroughly enamored with the Cascade Range, took it upon himself to impart his obsession to my brother and me. And so it was that I found myself beholding alpine meadows exploding into bloom from the safety of my dad's back before I could even walk the trails.

My earliest memories are all of mountains: riding the ski lift with my family in blizzard conditions, the smell of fir trees and lichen in our snow forts, the look on my grandpa's face when he encountered a bear, gorging myself on dark-blue huckleberries with my brother, being covered in mosquito bites, and listening to my grandma tell stories around the campfire. These experiences set the stage for my own passion for the outdoors and for all the wild things of this land.

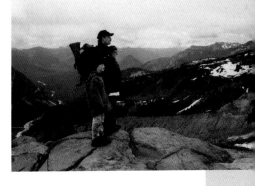

The Cascades are the centerpiece of the Pacific Northwest, but this diverse bioregion also includes deserts, rainforests, rugged coastlines, rain-shadowed islands, volcanoes, steppes, prairies, and more. Each ecosystem in this region hosts its own unique set of plants and animals.

Throughout my years of being totally obsessed with plants, I have had unique opportunities to see the important work that conservation groups do to protect our ecosystems, wildlife habitats and corridors, endemic plants, watersheds, threatened insects, and cultural landscapes. Through this, I have slowly come to understand the importance of human-driven stewardship and advocacy.

As a child, I saw the consequences of a nonreciprocal relationship with nature when I peered into collapsed mine shafts on Cougar Mountain and gazed out the car window at vast fields of clear-cuts out past Enumclaw. The first European settlers came to the Pacific Northwest to extract natural resources and send them elsewhere, a legacy that will be with us for many years to come. Something I have observed in my years teaching foraging is that most people who feel called to learn about wild plants are motivated by a deep craving to feel a connection to nature. We want to belong, and we cannot experience that sense of belonging by only taking.

Belonging stems from cultivating a reciprocal relationship with a community. It means receiving what can be received, and giving what can be given. It means considering the future abundance and health of the community in every action. Such a relationship is forged when a person takes the time to invest in the same land over a period of time. Year after year, showing up and coming to know the land where you live—this is my invitation to you.

Wild spaces are not just pristine mountaintops but also the cracks in the sidewalks, the weedy patch in the park, and the median strips in our neighborhoods. As you begin your journey into foraging, please enter all wild places with a sense of reverence and stewardship.

When I am harvesting with my students, there are moments when I feel a deep sense of rightness, like a puzzle piece clicking into place. Perhaps we are in silence, swishing through the grass to the next berry plant or chatting happily as we unearth a deep root from the ground with our hands. Foraging can be an act of reconnection to the land, and to our fellow humans.

It is my fervent belief that educating people about these special plants will create the advocates and stewards needed to protect our wild spaces. It is also my belief that having this knowledge is a kind of power. The power to have options when it comes to our health. The power to care for our friends and families.

My practice of using medicinal plants acknowledges and honors the knowledge that's come before. I live on Coast Salish land. The places noted in this book are all on Native land. The information in this book builds on knowledge and traditions that local Native groups have been practicing since time immemorial and continue to practice today. For my practice, I also draw heavily on the historical traditions of my own ancestors, who came to this continent from Ireland, England, Scotland, Norway, Denmark, and Sweden.

Introduction

Maybe you're new to herbal medicine. Maybe you're new to plant identification. Maybe you're new to being outside in general. No worries! This guide is designed to support both the beginner and intermediate herbalist. As with anything in life, start small and be consistent with your learning.

An herbalist is a person whose profession revolves around using plants for medicine. Within this field, there are people who see clients (clinical herbalists), people who make medicines for their community (community herbalists), people who harvest plants in the wild to sell (wildcrafters), herbal teachers, medicine makers, researchers, and lay herbalists (people who use herbs for themselves and their families but are not professional).

Every culture across the world has a tradition of healing with plants. Some examples of well-known traditions are Ayurveda, traditional Chinese medicine, plant spirit medicine, traditional Western herbalism, and Native North American herbal traditions. There are so many approaches, in fact, that you would be hard-pressed to find herbalists who have the exact same approach. My approach is a blend of traditional Western herbalism, Chinese herbalism, British folk herbalism, and my own discoveries. Herbalism is an invitation for you to discover what you believe and what kind of herbalist you want to be. My advice is to follow your curiosity.

This book will guide you in learning to forage for herbs and prepare herbal medicines. Part One covers the basics of identifying and harvesting wild plants and making medicine, and Part Two features specific plants and recipes to help you get started on this journey. Please supplement these with books, classes, and the internet. Different herbalists have different styles of medicine making, so it's good to learn from several sources to see what you like.

You will also learn how to use the plant medicines you prepare. This piece can take years to master, and you will still be learning even then. If you like falling down deep rabbit holes, you will love herbalism. You will learn about effective dosing, which preparations are best in a given scenario, how to select the right herbs for the job, and how to combine herbs effectively. Instead of starting with tackling a complex health issue, try starting with more simple scenarios. Things like putting pine resin salve on a paper cut, taking a willow bark tincture to relieve the pain from a sprained ankle, drinking mullein tea for a cough, or taking a cramp bark tincture for menstrual cramps are a few examples.

Finally, Part Three covers some of the most common poisonous and toxic plants to watch out for in the Pacific Northwest.

I am so excited for you to learn and explore. Most of all, I am excited for you to reunite with a tradition that is as old as time and to feel like a participant in the great cycles of nature. Be gentle with the plants, and be gentle with yourself.

Peeling the bark of chokecherry (*Prunus virginiana*) for use in a cough syrup (Photo by Vanessa Babida)

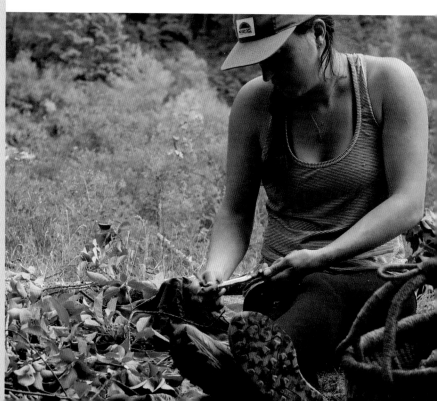

Safety

There are several safety concerns to keep in mind when using medicinal plants. Most importantly, pay attention to your body when taking herbs, and stop taking an herb if you experience any unpleasant side effects. For example, some herbs may cause dehydration or constipation. Herbs also have contraindications, which is a condition or situation in which you should not consume that herb. Pregnancy is the most common contraindication for herbs—there are many herbs that should not be consumed while pregnant. Watch for this note in "Cautions" sidebars throughout this book.

Herbs can also have negative interactions with pharmaceuticals. I note some contraindications and pharmaceutical interactions in the plant entries in Part Two, but they are not exhaustive. I encourage you to do your own research for personal safety, especially if you are currently taking any pharmaceuticals.

Also, some medicinal herbs are toxic in large doses. Though herbalists sometimes use toxic or poisonous plants, I recommend experimenting with the more toxic plants only after studying for several years. I note the toxicity in the Cautions sidebar at the end of each plant entry in Part Two. Of the thirty-five herbs featured in this book, the only one with considerable toxicity is Pacific bleeding heart (*Dicentra formosa*), and the toxicity concerns are thoroughly outlined in that plant's listing. Most medicinal herbs should not be consumed in large doses, as you would an edible plant. For example, Oregon grape bark, cedar leaves, and elderberries are commonly used medicinal herbs, but these contain compounds that could hurt you if taken in very large doses. Notes are included in each of those entries to help you better understand the risks associated with each plant. Refer to Part Three for detailed information about local poisonous and toxic plants to avoid while foraging.

Cautions

Pay close attention to these Cautions sidebars for warnings about specific contraindications for each plant.

Part One

Learn to Forage for Herbs and Make Medicine

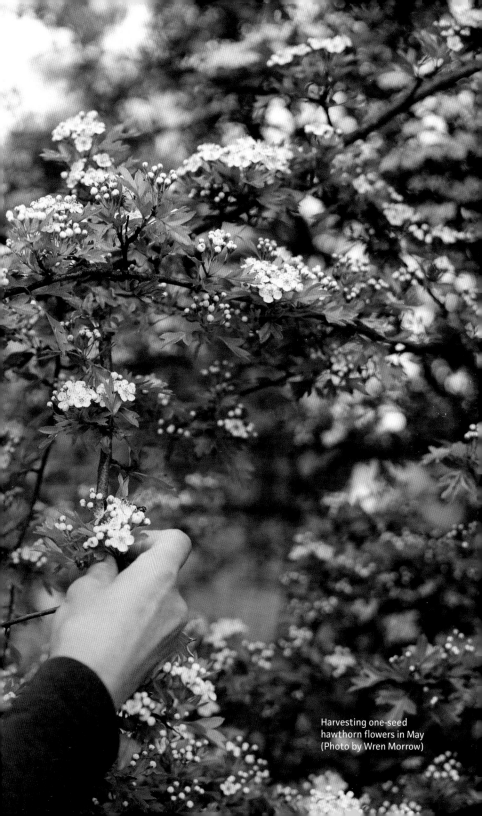

Harvesting one-seed
hawthorn flowers in May
(Photo by Wren Morrow)

This section covers the basic skills needed to choose harvesting spots, harvest respectfully, develop your plant ID skills and knowledge, harvest plants at the right time, and have the right equipment on hand. I recommend that beginner foragers peruse this section before heading out for the first time. Intermediate foragers will find valuable reference material in this section, and perhaps some new ideas about stewardship.

Harvesting Medicinal Plants

Harvesting is a skill in and of itself, one that is not well represented in many guides. A successful harvest outing depends on knowing what equipment you will need, where to go, when to go, what part of the plant to harvest, how much to harvest, and how to process it when you get home. Use the information in this book as your starting point, then add to your knowledge by learning more from experienced harvesters and through your own observation and direct experiences.

It's also important to consider how your actions will affect the plants, the local ecosystem, and wildlife. The impact of harvesting medicinal plants in wild spaces can be ecologically devastating or ecologically beneficial. I invite you to strive toward maximum ecological benefit in your harvests, and I have provided further recommendations on this topic in the Harvesting for the Health of Our Ecosystems section. The best place to start is to harvest what's abundant, which is why I chose the most common plants to feature in this book. Some of these plants are considered native, which means they occur naturally and were not introduced by humans. Some are non-native, also known as exotic species or introduced species. These plants were introduced by humans to the ecosystem, where they became naturalized, meaning that they grow spontaneously without human intervention.

Developing Your Plant ID Skills

Plant identification is one of the most difficult skills to learn, and the most critical. Before you put anything in your mouth, make sure your ID is 100 percent correct. The same species of a plant can differ in color, size, and shape depending on where it's growing and the time of year. Learning to note small details like hairs on the stem, serrations on the leaf edge, the shape of the flowers, the inflorescence (the arrangement of flowers along the axis of the stem), and where the plant is growing will help you immensely on your identification journey. Plant identification apps and plant identification forums can be helpful too, though keep in mind that there is a margin for error in both. Here are several strategies you can use to get better acquainted with local plants:

- Go outside and spend time looking at plants. Get curious about them.
- Take an in-person class out in the field.
- Use plant identification apps on your phone (but don't trust them 100 percent).
- Use social media plant identification forums (but don't trust them 100 percent).
- Buy local field guides.
- Use the internet (YouTube, podcasts, blogs, etc.).
- Learn about plant families and taxonomy.

Scientific Names and Taxonomy

Plant taxonomy is the study of how plants are related and categorized. All living organisms can be categorized using the Linnaean system (named after the Swedish botanist Carolus Linnaeus). It helps immensely to know a bit about the classifications of plants and their Latin names as you learn to identify plants. Though this book deals almost exclusively with species in the plant kingdom, one entry falls outside the plant kingdom: usnea lichen, which is a fungus with an algal symbiont (meaning an algae that is in a symbiotic relationship with the fungus, exchanging functions to support one another).

The levels of classification are summed up in the hierarchical chart on page 18, starting with the largest categories and ending with the most specific.

Herbalists and foragers are most concerned with the last three lines of the chart: family, genus, and species. The plant family is a larger group of many plants that share similarities in flower type and DNA because they have the same ancestors. For example, several plants in this book are in the rose family, such as blackberry and rose. They share certain characteristics, but without

a trained eye, you might not know they are related. Families are composed of genera (the plural form of *genus*). A genus is a smaller grouping of related species within a family that can often look quite similar. Some entries in this book will contain two or more plants in the same genus, such as broadleaf plantain (*Plantago major*) and narrowleaf plantain (*Plantago lanceolata*), which are both in the plantain genus (*Plantago*). A species is a single, genetically distinct organism that typically cannot mate with other species (though there are exceptions to this).

The classic two-part botanical name that you will see throughout this book is called a Latin binomial, such as *Arctostaphylos uva-ursi*. The name contains the genus (first word) and species (second word). Let's take a look at an example of the botanical names found in this book:

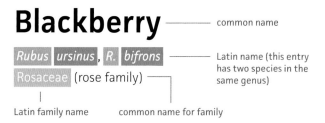

Blackberry —————— common name

Rubus *ursinus*, *R.* *bifrons* ———— Latin name (this entry
has two species in the
same genus)

Rosaceae (rose family) ——┐

│   │

Latin family name   common name for family

You might be asking why you should bother with all of this technical information. Though it isn't required to know to go out and forage, knowing about plant families and plant taxonomy in general can be helpful for a few key reasons:

- If you know by sight what family a plant is in, identifying it will be much easier. Many field guides are organized by family.

- Knowing how plants are related can help you predict and remember their medicinal uses. The rose family, for example, tends to contain a lot of astringent compounds and flavonoids.
- Having a structural framework to organize information makes it easier to remember. This system has helped me remember a large number of plants by organizing them into groups in my head.
- In some cases, very similar species may be rarer or less medicinal than the species you want to harvest. Beginner foragers often harvest these look-alikes by accident. The more you understand the specific distinctions between species and familiarize yourself with resources that help with identification, the less likely you are to accidentally harvest the wrong plant.
- You will better understand more advanced sources, such as floras (technical books that list all the plant species of a given location), scientific articles, and essays.

Start by simply taking note of the scientific names in this book. Say them out loud and notice Latin roots that you may recognize.

Preparing to Harvest

Before you head out into the field, make sure you have a plan for harvesting, processing, and using the herb you intend to forage: Know what you will use the plant for and how much you need. Know where to harvest the plant, what part of the plant to harvest, and when (see Timing Your Harvest).

Where to Go

Choosing good harvest spots can be tricky. The safest and most reliable place to harvest is in your own yard or on the land of someone you know. Public lands can often be a good place to harvest, though be aware that there are sometimes rules and restrictions, or a license may be required to harvest there.

Harvesting regulations for public land depend on how the land is classified (e.g., city park, county park, state park, preserve, wilderness area, national park, National Forest Service, Bureau of Land Management, Department of Natural

Resources). There are typically different requirements for personal harvest and commercial harvest. Certain areas may require getting a license only for commercial harvesting; others may require a license for personal harvesting also. Some areas will not allow any harvesting at all, and others may specify what plant parts or species may be gathered there. Some trailheads and parks will have signs that specifically say "no harvesting." Each municipality will have different rules, so you will need to look them up for your specific area.

Harvesting on private land, on the other hand, is much simpler: you just need permission from the landowner. I have some friends who own land and allow me to harvest there. Sometimes I ask organic farms if I can harvest some of their weeds, like lambsquarters, plantain, and pineapple weed. Facebook, Buy Nothing groups, and other online forums are great places to ask neighbors and friends if they have certain plants that you can harvest.

Regardless of where you harvest, be sure to avoid areas with pesticides, fecal matter, and other contaminants. This could include roadsides, dog parks, old mines, areas around telephone poles, and recent construction sites.

The seed heads of western pasqueflower and various species of heather in flower in Mount Rainier National Park (Photo by Julien Bacon)

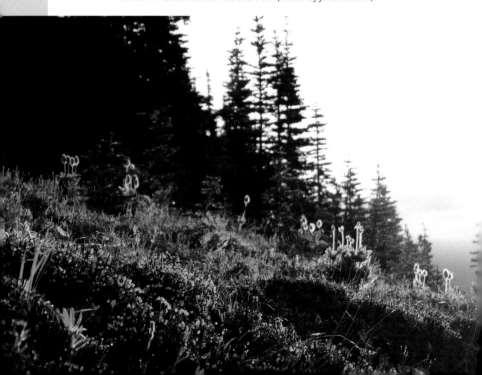

What to Bring

Use sharp, clean tools for harvesting. Clean tools help prevent the spread of disease, and sharp tools reduce the surface area opened up when you cut, reducing the disease vector. Here is a list of all the tools I use for foraging, ranked from most used to least used in the field:

- clippers
- scissors
- paper, fabric, or mesh bags (preferable over plastic because of mold)
- rubber-coated gardening gloves
- thick leather gardening gloves (for harvesting spiny or thorned plants, like blackberry)
- pocketknife
- hori-hori knife (a Japanese digging knife)
- butter knife
- four-pronged digging fork (for digging up roots)
- scrub brush (for scrubbing the dirt off roots or lichen and moss off branches)
- folding handsaw
- loppers (for cutting larger branches)
- parchment-paper bags (for harvesting resin)
- jeweler's loupe (a type of magnifying glass)
- a pickax (for digging larger roots in rocky soil)

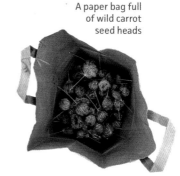

A paper bag full of wild carrot seed heads

When you get home, hose any dirt off your tools and let them dry before storing.

If you are going to a more remote location to harvest, consider what clothing, gear, and food you might need. Foraging is slightly different from hiking, as you often leave the established trail, which means that you are more likely to encounter brambles, insects, wildlife, uneven ground, and other hazards. Here is a short list of additional things to consider bringing along:

- sturdy hiking shoes (not sandals, so you don't get poked or stung)

- long pants (to protect your legs from getting scratched by brambles, or from getting ticks)
- snacks and lunch
- at least 1 liter of water, or 2 for a longer day
- rain jacket
- warm jacket and hat
- cell phone or other communication device (as there is often no cell service in the wilderness)
- backpack (preferably one with a hip belt)
- map of the area
- brightly colored clothing or even a reflective vest (if harvesting in an area where people hunt)

Always exercise caution when out in remote areas. There are many potential hazards, including wildlife, hunters, unexpected weather, cliffs, rivers, and more. Avoid going out alone, and always inform someone of where you will be and when to expect you back. When leaving an established trail, do not go far without proper training in navigation and a map of the area. It is common for foragers to get lost in the woods.

Harvesting for the Health of Our Ecosystems

As the climate changes and our wild spaces diminish, and as foraging gets more popular, we must be more and more careful with how we forage. Popular plants such as Solomon's seal, echinacea, and American ginseng have long been overharvested. Native plants, especially those plants that have specialized habitats, are also continually threatened by agriculture, changes in wildfire patterns, invasive species, timber harvest, and development. The South Puget Sound prairies, a bioregion-specific ecosystem that I studied in college, have been greatly reduced since this area was colonized. Many plants are disappearing altogether as their habitats recede or are fragmented by development. Great work is being done by conservation groups to protect remaining habitat, remove invasive species, increase the populations of threatened species, and do much-needed research. As foragers, we can do our part by respecting sensitive habitats and getting educated on what plant populations are declining.

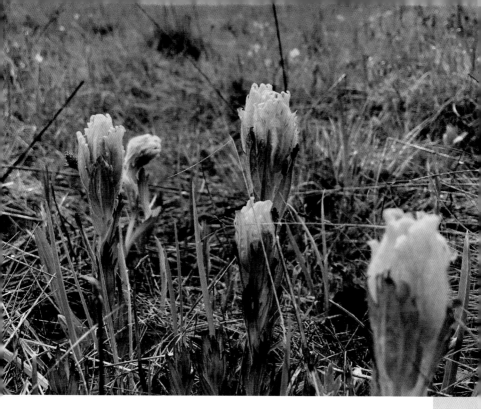

Golden paintbrush (*Castilleja levisecta*), an endemic prairie plant, growing at Glacial Heritage Preserve near Olympia, Washington

When foraging, we can diligently observe the relative abundance of the species we harvest year after year and change our harvesting practices based on what we see. There are many practices medicinal plant foragers can adopt, including selective pruning, seed dispersal by hand, invasive species removal (such as ivy and blackberries), and replanting root eyes. We can also avoid harvesting rare plants altogether and limit our harvest of less abundant plants. Here are some essential principles to follow every time you forage:

- Avoid harvesting the first plant you see. Practice patience and observe how abundant the plant actually is and whether there is a larger, healthier stand nearby.
- Harvest for maximum future growth. For example, thin plants where they are crowded, or replant the root eyes elsewhere. This book offers tips on how to do this for specific plants.

- Harvest one in ten, which means that you should harvest no more than one out of every ten plants you see. This rule may differ slightly by plant.
- Look for signs of others' harvesting—look for cut stems or holes—and alter your harvest accordingly.
- Leave some flowers to go to seed. Leave some fruits for birds and other animals.

Once, hiking through a field of osha (*Ligusticum* spp.) in the North Cascades, I sat to watch the chipmunks, who would reach up to the seed heads and use their tiny paws to pick the seeds off

Chocolate lily (*Fritillaria affinis*), growing at Glacial Heritage Preserve in an area where prescribed burning is being reintroduced. Low-intensity burns help some food plants like this thrive.

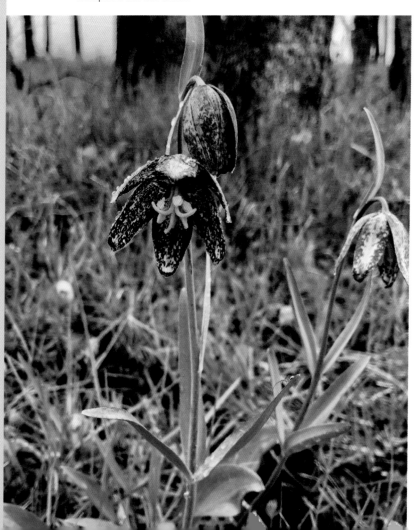

and shove them into their cheeks until they were bursting. It is easy to not think about how other species might need the thing we are harvesting if we can't see it happening. Maybe we show up at a different time of year, and not on the frigid January day when the flock of cedar waxwings come to eat the last berries of one-seeded hawthorn (*Crataegus monogyna*). One way that I like to ensure that I am leaving enough for everyone is to follow the grazing patterns of a deer. A deer will munch a leaf, then go to the next tree and munch some leaves from that tree, and then go on to the next tree. When I forage, I take some berries from one bush, some from the next, and so forth.

The most powerful way to act in harmony with the ecosystems you encounter is to develop a relationship with the places you harvest from. Here are some suggestions for deepening your relationship with the spots you visit to harvest:

- Observe closely. Visit several times a year to observe the land in different seasons. What animals are there? What insects?
- Go to the same spots and note what is changing year after year. Are stands getting smaller? Are there more fruits one year and fewer the next? Do the flowers bloom at the same time every year?
- Learn the history of that land and the surrounding areas. What Native group traditionally tended it? Has it been logged or mined? Was it once a farm?
- Take note of the plants nearby. Are there sensitive plants? Are there invasive species? If there are sensitive species around, take care not to tread on them or impact them with your harvest.

Timing Your Harvest

Knowing exactly when to harvest something is one of the most elusive and key skills of a forager. English hawthorn (*Crataegus monogyna*), for example, blooms for one week each year. Not only that, but its flowers are best harvested right as they open, when some flowers are still buds. That means there may be a four-to-six-day window in the year to harvest it at its best! There are a number of approaches you can take to ensure you roll in to your patch during prime time:

- Take pictures on your smartphone every year so you can remember what bloomed when each year. Smartphone pictures have date stamps that you can use as reference.
- Follow local foragers on social media and see what they are posting.
- Pay attention to what's happening with the plants on the medians and the sides of the freeway. Roads create a warmer microclimate, which means that bloom times there are slightly earlier. If hawthorn is blooming next to the freeway, it will soon bloom at your local spot.
- Put harvest windows on your calendar to plan in advance (see Seasonal Harvest Calendar), and record when you harvested what on your calendar.

Regardless of the specific plant you intend to harvest, it's best to avoid harvesting in damp weather. If you cannot avoid it, tincture immediately, or use a heat source for drying. In addition, early morning is the best time to harvest, when volatile oils are the highest. The afternoon on a hot, sunny day is the worst.

Factors That Affect Timing

The temperatures and frosts between February and April affect when plants leaf out and bloom. Sometimes we have an early year, when there is warmer weather in early spring, and sometimes we have a late cold snap in March or even April that pushes back the bloom times.

Elevation is also a huge factor in when things bloom. Red elder (*Sambucus racemosa*) blooms around March at sea level and as late as July in the Cascades at 4,000 feet and above. Stinging nettle (*Urtica dioica*) is typically ready to harvest at sea level around the Puget Sound in February, but if you go up even 300 feet in elevation, it may not be ready yet.

Cities create their own heat, which means that more populated areas will bloom earlier than the countryside surrounding them, even if they are at the same elevation.

Guidelines for Timing the Harvest of Specific Plant Parts

Your timing will also vary depending on what part of the plant you intend to harvest. Some basic guidelines for different plant parts are provided here, and you can also use the Seasonal

Harvest Calendar to look up the harvesting window for specific plant parts.

ROOTS

Perennial roots, such as dandelion and yellow dock, are typically harvested when the leafy parts aboveground are dead or dying. This is when the energy is in the roots. In our climate, this means in the fall or spring. As for harvesting roots in winter: If the ground is frozen, it's hard to dig. However, the ground does not freeze much west of the Cascades, so winter harvest can be possible too. The exact timing varies depending on how early the first frost is and the particular plant.

The one downside to harvesting roots when the aerial parts are dead and dying is that it can be more difficult to identify and even find the plants. This is where your summer observations come in handy. Spot the plants with roots you want to harvest early and come back in the fall. You can even drop a pin on Google Maps and set a reminder on your phone!

Western pasqueflower (*Anemone occidentalis*) emerging just after the snow has melted in Mount Rainier National Park. These subalpine and alpine habitats are some of the most sensitive. (Photo by Julien Bacon)

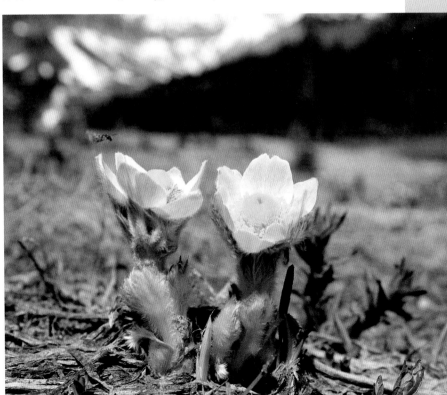

BARK

Bark is also harvested in spring or fall. Spring bark is wetter and sweeter and can be easier to peel because of the higher water content. Willow (*Salix* spp.) bark is nice to harvest in March because it peels off in large sheets. Bark harvested in the fall is a bit drier and more acrid.

I am an opportunistic bark scavenger: I harvest when the neighbors trim their trees or after a windstorm. I once encountered a pile of tall, freshly cut Oregon grape branches on a walk in my neighborhood, and the city landscapers happily told me to take as much as I wanted. I think I made a half gallon of Oregon grape tincture that day!

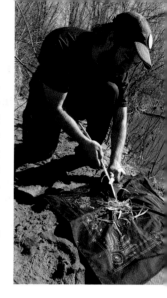

Harvesting willow bark on the banks of the Green River in February. Barks are typically harvested before the leaves emerge in the spring.

FLOWERS

Flowers are always best to harvest when they have just opened, with some even still in bud. For example, St. John's wort (*Hypericum perforatum*) flowers are most potent when they are just about to open.

FRUITS AND SEEDS

Seeds and fruits ripen at different times depending on the plant. Most will be ripe in late summer. Note that some seeds are best harvested when mature, and some seeds, such as wild carrot, should be harvested when immature. Berries and other fleshy fruits should always be harvested at peak ripeness.

LEAVES

Leaves have the most highly variable timing of any of the plant parts. The key is to harvest when the leaves are the most vibrant. For edible plants, the young plants are typically the best, as is the case with stinging nettle (*Urtica dioica*) and chickweed (*Stellaria media*), but that isn't necessarily true of medicinal plants. As leaves get older, they often produce more secondary compounds, which are what we use for medicine. Find more specific guidance on when to harvest leaves in the individual plant entries in Part Two.

Processing Your Harvest

After a day of foraging in the wild, there is often much to do. Perhaps you have harvested four or more different plants and need to peel, pluck, and tincture. Factor this processing time into your day when harvesting, and avoid harvesting more than you have time to process; many plants go to waste when people don't account for the processing time. Here are some tips on processing and storing both fresh and dried plant material:

- Rinse dirty roots with a hose immediately upon arriving home. Afterward, scrub with a stiff-bristled scrub brush in a bucket of water. Sometimes I scrub roots out in the field if I can find a clean stream nearby.
- Strip bark branches as soon as possible; every day you wait, the task will become more difficult. With the blade pointing away from you, use a knife to peel the bark into a basket or onto a cloth.
- Try to avoid washing leaves and flowers with water as it can ruin your chances of drying and may diminish the plant's medicine.
- If you notice a lot of bugs in your harvest, give them time to crawl out by putting the bag with your harvest on its side for a few hours outside. Also be aware that bugs may crawl out of the bags into your car while you are driving. I have had to pull over many times on the way home to escort spiders out of the car.

Spraying the dirt off a recently harvested yellow dock root with a garden hose

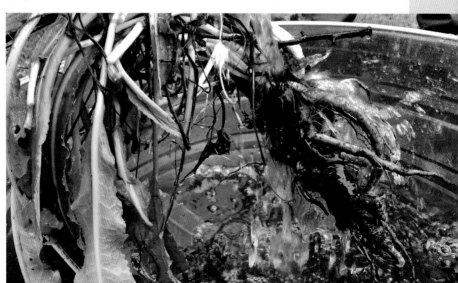

SEASONAL HARVEST CALENDAR

PLANT	JAN	FEB	MAR
Black cottonwood buds	■	■	
Blackberry berry			
Blackberry root	▨	▨	■
Bleeding heart (whole plant in flower)			▨
Blue elderberry			
Blue elderflower			
California poppy (whole plant in flower)			
Chickweed	▨		■
Cleavers			■
Cramp bark	■	■	■
Dandelion leaf	▨	▨	
Dandelion root	■	■	■
Douglas-fir resin	■	■	■
Douglas-fir tips			
Fir tips			
Goldenrod leaf and flower			
Gumweed buds			
Hawthorn berry (black)			
Hawthorn berry (one-seed)			
Hawthorn leaf and flower (all species)			
Horsetail vegetative shoots			
Mugwort leaf			
Mullein flower			
Mullein leaf			■
Oregon grape bark	■	■	■

■ Ideal time to harvest.

▨ Shoulder season. Available but not ideal.
Look to higher elevations or microclimates.

APR	MAY	JUN	JUL	AUG	SEP	OCT	NOV	DEC
						▨		▨
			▨	■				
▨	▨	▨				■	■	▨
■	■							
					▨	▨		
	■	■						
		▨	▨	▨				
■						■	■	▨
■								
						■	■	■
▨	▨	▨				■	■	■
▨	■	■	■	■	■	■	■	■
	■	■						
		■						
		▨	■	■				
	▨	■	■					
		▨	■					
						■		
	■							
■								
	■	■						
	▨	■	■	■				
▨	▨	▨	▨	▨				
▨	▨	▨	▨	▨	▨	■	■	■

SEASONAL HARVEST CALENDAR

PLANT	JAN	FEB	MAR
Oregon grape berry			
Pine resin	■	■	■
Plantain husks and seeds			
Plantain leaf			▨
Red clover flower			
Red elderberry			
Red elderflower			■
Red root (root bark)			
Rose hips			
Rose petals			
Spruce tips			
St. John's wort buds and flowers			
Stinging nettle leaf		▨	■
Stinging nettle root	▨	■	■
Stinging nettle seed			
Usnea thallus	■	■	▨
Uva ursi leaf	■	■	■
Violet flower	▨	■	■
Violet leaf	▨	■	■
Western redcedar leaf	▨	▨	▨
Wild carrot (green seed head)			
Wild carrot flower			
Willow bark	■	■	■
Yarrow flowering tops			
Yellow dock root	■	■	■

Ideal time to harvest.

Shoulder season. Available but not ideal.
Look to higher elevations or microclimates.

APR	MAY	JUN	JUL	AUG	SEP	OCT	NOV	DEC

Storing Fresh Plant Material

Fresh plants that can't be made into medicine right away should be kept in the fridge, ideally for not more than three days. After that, either make medicine or dry them (see Tips for Drying). If it was raining when you harvested, don't wait to process, as plant material is more likely to mold during storage.

Certain fresh plants will degrade more quickly than others, such as St. John's wort, arnica, and albizzia flower. They shouldn't be stored for long, if at all. Other items, like berries, buds, and barks, can be frozen for later use.

Drying Plant Material

Most of the Pacific Northwest is quite moist, so you will need to take extra care when drying plant material to prevent mold.

- Avoid exposure to sunlight. It is a common misconception that drying things in the sun is a good idea. The sun certainly dries things fast, but it also damages a lot of constituents.
- Dry on a porous surface. Paper, natural fiber fabric, baskets, and drying racks made specifically for drying plant material all work. These surfaces absorb extra condensation, unlike metal or plastic.
- Spread the material out as much as possible. If you end up with a lot of overlapping, simply stir and turn over the plant material once a day to allow air to access all pieces.
- Leave on the drying rack until very dry. To test, crush some in your hand. It should break easily and be crunchy. Some plants dry more quickly than others, so there is no strict timeline for drying.
- Cut up fleshy plant parts. Roots, fleshy stems, and thick flower buds can all be sliced in half or cut up to dry more quickly, reducing the risk of mold.
- Check frequently by smell and sight. If you do find mold, remove the affected plants immediately to prevent the mold from spreading.
- Invest in a dehydrator if you continue to have trouble with mold. Some houses are more mold-prone than others. I have never owned a dehydrator and never have had a problem, but I have talked to folks who live in damp homes who have had trouble drying their herbs without them molding.

Processing and Storing Dried Plant Material

Once your plants are dry, it is time to garble and store. To garble something is to tear off the leaves and break it down into smaller pieces to make it easy to use later. For example, when you harvest and dry thyme on woody stems, remove the leaves once they are dry. For fennel seed, remove the dried seeds from the seed head before storing. I love to garble on the living room floor while watching a good movie.

Store dried herbs in glass jars if possible. Glass jars offer the best balance between moisture control and bug control. You can also store in paper or plastic bags, but keep in mind that it's common for insects to get into bags of dried herbs. If you see new holes, webs, larvae, or living bugs in a bag of herbs, throw it out immediately. And because plastic traps in moisture, be sure to dry plants thoroughly before storing them in plastic bags. Label your dried herbs with the name of the plant, the plant part, the harvest date, and the location of harvest.

Dried herbs lose their potency the longer they are stored, and their shelf life varies depending on the specific plant and plant part. I keep dried herbs anywhere from one to four years. Flowers tend to last the shortest amount of time and should be kept for only one to two years. Roots and berries can be kept for longer. Aging herbs begin to lose their color and smell, and should be composted at that point. If it still smells nice and the color is good, then it is probably still okay to use. Increase the shelf life of your herbs by keeping them in a dark, cool, dry place.

Removing the leaves from dried mugwort stems

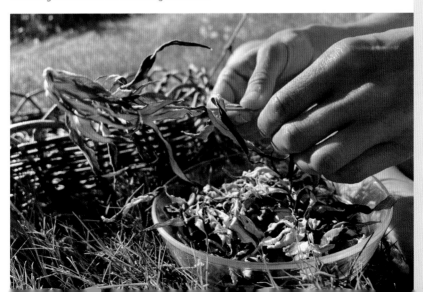

Making Medicine

Preparing herbal medicines is an essential skill for any herbalist, especially one who is harvesting their own medicinal plants. This section focuses on the two most common preparations: tinctures and teas. There are a number of other preparations featured in the recipes, such as oxymels, cordials, and infused vinegars, along with detailed instructions on how to prepare them. Find descriptions of these in the Other Preparations section at the end of this chapter.

Tinctures

A tincture is an alcohol extract of a medicinal plant. To make one, you soak the plant in alcohol for about a month, strain it, and dispense it into a little dropper bottle. Tinctures are very shelf stable and are easy to carry around and use. They can be used both internally and topically—tinctures for topical use are called liniments.

The dosage of many tinctures taken internally is 30 to 60 drops. When experimenting with tinctures, always start with the smallest dose and work up from there. Some people may be sensitive or allergic to particular plants, or they may simply need a lower dose of it. Note also that some medicinal plants are slightly toxic. We call these low-dose plants, and they are taken in smaller doses to avoid adverse side effects.

Because tinctures are made with strong alcohol, some people like to take them with a bit of water. To avoid diluting them too much, take with no more than an ounce of water.

Understanding and Using Ratios

Understanding ratios is a foundational element of making herbal medicines because ratios allow us to make scalable recipes. We use them in herbalism to make products of consistent concentration. A ratio is listed as two numbers separated by a colon, such as 1:1 or 1:7.

A standardized tincture is one made using a ratio. A folk tincture is one made without measurements, using the eyeball method. I make standardized tinctures for many plants because the potency is more consistent and predictable.

In this book, I use imperial measurements: ounces for weight measurements and fluid ounces for volume measurements. I recommend getting a digital kitchen scale and some accurate glass measuring cups.

The liquid solvent used in the tincturing process is called the menstruum and is typically alcohol. When making tinctures with dried plant material, I typically use a 1:5 ratio, which means for every 1 ounce of dried plant material, I will add 5 fluid ounces of alcohol.

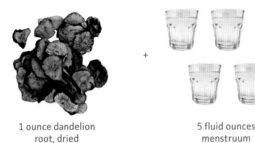

1 ounce dandelion root, dried   5 fluid ounces menstruum

Now let's use the ratio to scale up. Say that I have 5 ounces of dried dandelion root that I want to tincture. Multiply that by 5, and I get 25 fluid ounces of menstruum needed.

For making tinctures with fresh plant material, I often use a 1:2 ratio. This ratio indicates that for every 1 ounce of plant material, I will use 2 fluid ounces of alcohol.

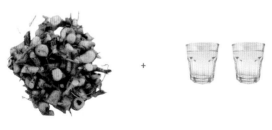

1 ounce dandelion root, fresh   2 fluid ounces menstruum

For example, if I have 4.5 ounces of fresh dandelion root, I need to multiply the amount of plant material by 2 (the second number in the ratio) to get the amount of alcohol, so in my jar, I'll put 4.5 ounces of fresh dandelion root and 9 fluid ounces of alcohol.

There are exceptions to these standard ratios, however. Some plants are much less dense than others, which means they will need more alcohol and a higher ratio. For example, mullein is so light and fluffy that I use a 1:20 ratio for the dried leaf. Use the Tincture Ratio Chart to find out what ratio and alcohol percentage to use for each plant in the book.

Deciding to Use Fresh or Dry Plant Material

Some plants can be tinctured fresh or dry (like dandelion root), some need to be tinctured fresh (like St. John's wort), and others need to be tinctured dry (like cramp bark). For plants that must be dried first, it is usually because there is an undesirable compound that gets reduced through drying. For plants that must be tinctured fresh, there are typically important medicinal compounds that degrade in the drying process. The Tincture Ratio Chart includes ratios for both fresh and dried plant material, except when it's not advisable to make medicine from the fresh or dried plant. Where there is a choice, I often end up using plants that have been recently dried for many tinctures.

Maximizing Extraction by Increasing Surface Area

Over the years I have rediscovered, again and again, the simple power of breaking down the plant material before extraction. This allows the menstruum (alcohol, vinegar, honey, etc.) to access more surface area, which maximizes opportunities for extracting compounds from the plant.

For dried plants, I use an electric grinder to grind up the plant material into the consistency of coarse sand. For fresh plants, I use a blender to puree the plant material with the alcohol to make a smoothie-like sludge. You can also chop the plant finely with a knife. Some plants, like barks and roots, are more difficult to break down because they are so woody.

When choosing an electric grinder, keep in mind that coffee grinders are made to grind coffee beans and often cannot handle some of the woody plant material that herbalists like to grind. I broke the first coffee grinder I ever got on its first day of use by trying to grind dried roots. Since then I have always purchased spice-and-nut grinders, which are slightly more sturdy. Also, the smell of coffee pervades anything it touches and will make your herbal preparations taste and smell like coffee if you use your grinder for both. I recommend getting a separate grinder to use for your herbs.

Selecting the Alcohol Percentage

Each entry in the Tincture Ratio Chart indicates what percentage of alcohol to use for that specific plant. Some entries recommend different percentages for different plant parts, or a different recommendation if the plant is fresh versus dry. Note that alcohol percentage is *not* the same as the proof of the alcohol. Everclear, for example, is 190 proof but 95 percent alcohol.

Measuring alcohol to make a standardized tincture

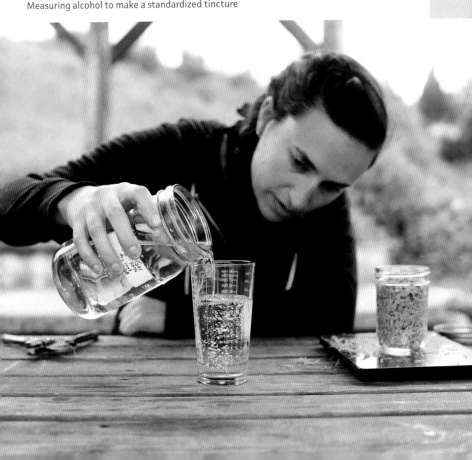

You'll need to use a higher alcohol percentage (90 percent to 100 percent alcohol) for resins and resinous plants, which are insoluble in water. For aromatic plants and plants with primarily alcohol-soluble constituents, use 60 percent to 80 percent alcohol. For plants that are not aromatic or resinous, 40 percent to 50 percent alcohol is perfect. It is common to use a higher alcohol concentration for tincturing fresh plants because they add their own water to the solution. You can dilute Everclear to create any percentage of alcohol you like. (Note: In some states, you need a license to buy Everclear.)

I typically use vodka (either 40 percent or 50 percent alcohol by volume) or Everclear (95 percent alcohol by volume) for tincture making. Some people like to use brandy, rum, and other types of alcohol for their tinctures, but I avoid these because I prefer not to have any preexisting flavors interfere with the plant's taste so that I can assess how strong the tincture is and what flavors are present. If you like to use organic alcohol, you can buy pure organic cane alcohol in bulk online (see Resources).

For certain plants, adding 10 percent vegetable glycerin to the alcohol tincture is recommended. When saponins and tannins coexist in the same solution, they react and create a globby precipitate at the bottom of the tincture. Adding a bit of vegetable glycerin can help stabilize the solution and prevent this. Of the plants in this book, this is recommended for yellow dock root, red root, hawthorn, cramp bark, and blackberry root.

Letting It Macerate

Tinctures are traditionally left to macerate for four weeks. You can shake it a few times during that period, partly to facilitate extraction and partly to prevent oxidation and mold if there are parts of the plant sticking into the air. That said, I rarely see tinctures grow mold.

If you let your tincture sit for longer than a month, check for signs of mold filaments on the exposed plant material. If you find signs of mold, discard the tincture. If you don't see any mold, it's fine to strain and use the tincture. I often let tinctures macerate for many months and have never had a problem.

DOUBLE MACERATION

Double maceration is a method used to make stronger tinctures by using two batches of herbs. You first make a regular tincture, let it macerate, and strain it. Then you add a new batch of plant material to the same alcohol and let it sit for another four weeks. As noted above, higher-proof alcohol is usually needed when tincturing fresh plants because the water from the plants dilutes the alcohol. This is especially true when using multiple batches of plant material, as that also means twice the water. I use the double-maceration method mostly for herbs that are extremely fluffy and thus hard to get a strong ratio with, like mullein leaf.

Straining Tinctures

To strain tinctures and other extractions, drape a piece of cheesecloth, a piece of cotton bedsheet, or a nut-milk bag over a fine-mesh strainer, and set the strainer atop a glass measuring cup. After adding the herbs to the top, gather up the cloth and squeeze the excess liquid out of the plant material. Sometimes you can wash the cloth and reuse it, but for oils or strong-tasting plants, it's best to toss it.

TINCTURE RATIO CHART

Plant	Plant part	Fresh ratio and alcohol percentage	Dry ratio and alcohol percentage	Notes
Black cottonwood	buds	1:2 or 1:3 at 95%	—	
Blackberry	root	1:2 at 75%	1:5 at 50%	add 10% glycerin
Bleeding heart	whole plant in flower	1:2 or 1:3 at 75%	1:5 or 1:6 at 50–60%	toxic in large doses
California poppy	whole plant in flower	1:3 or 1:4 at 75%	1:5 or 1:6 at 50–60%	
Cleavers	aerial parts before flowering	1:3 at 50%	—	A more typical preparation is a succus (a plant juice preserved with alcohol); see recipe in Cleavers entry
Cramp bark	bark	—	1:5 at 50%	add 10% glycerin

Plant	Plant part	Fresh ratio and alcohol percentage	Dry ratio and alcohol percentage	Notes
Dandelion	root	1:2 at 60–70%	1:5 at 50%	
Douglas-fir	resin	1:2 at 95%	—	
Douglas-fir	tips	1:3 at 50–75%	—	
Elder, blue	berry	1:2 at 50–60%	1:5 at 50%	
Elder, blue	flower	1:2 or 1:3 at 75%	1:5 at 50–60%	
Elder, red	flower	1:2 or 1:3 at 75%	1:5 at 50–60%	
Fir	tips	1:3 at 50–75%	—	
Goldenrod	flowers	1:2 or 1:3 at 75%	—	
Gumweed	resinous buds	1:2 or 1:3 at 95%	—	
Hawthorn	berry	—	1:5 at 50%	add 10% glycerin
Hawthorn	flowers	1:2 or 1:3 at 50–60%	1:5 or 1:6 at 50%	add 10% glycerin
Horsetail	green shoots	—	1.5 or 1:6 at 40%	fresh plant is toxic
Mugwort	leaf	1:3 or 1:4 at 75%	1:6 or 1:7 at 50–60%	
Mullein	leaf	—	1:20 at 40–50%	recommend double maceration
Mullein	root	1:2 at 60%	1:5 at 50%	
Oregon grape	stem bark	1:3 or 1:4 at 60%	1:5 at 40% to 50%	
Pine	resin	1:2 at 95%	—	
Plantain	leaf	1:2 at 60–75%	1:5 at 50%	
Red clover	flower	1:3 at 60–75%	1:6 at 40–50%	
Red root	root bark	1:2 at 75%	—	add 10% glycerin

Plant	Plant part	Fresh ratio and alcohol percentage	Dry ratio and alcohol percentage	Notes
Rose	hips	1:2 at 50–60%	1:5 at 50%	
Rose	petals	—	1:5 at 60%	
Spruce	tips	1:3 at 50–75%	—	
St. John's wort	buds and flowers	1:2 or 1:3 at 75%	—	
Stinging nettle	leaf	1:2 at 75%	1:4 at 50%	
Stinging nettle	root	1:2 at 75%	1:5 at 50–60%	
Stinging nettle	seed	—	1:5 at 50–60%	
Usnea	thallus	—	double extract	see recipe in Usnea entry
Uva ursi	leaf	—	1:5 at 50–60%	
Western redcedar	leaf	1:2 at 75%	1:5 at 60%	
Wild carrot	immature green seed heads	1:3 at 75%	1:5 or 1:6 at 50–60%	
Willow	bark	1:2 or 1:3 at 60%	1:5 at 50%	
Yarrow	flowering tops	1:2 at 75%	1:5 at 75%	
Yellow dock	root	1:2 at 70%	1:5 at 60%	add 10% glycerin

Herbal Teas

A tea is known as an infusion because it is made by steeping, or infusing, plant material—usually dry—in either cold or hot water. Infusions are the safest and most gentle herbal preparation. Though water is not as strong a solvent as alcohol for some constituents, it does not cause inflammation like alcohol does.

Hot infusions work best for flowers and leaves, whereas harder plant parts are best boiled in a preparation known as a decoction. Cold infusions are best for specific plants with heat-sensitive compounds.

There are many tea formulas among the recipes in Part Two that blend different dried herbs measured by weight. When formulating tea blends, I consider both medicinal actions and flavor. Feel free to tweak the recipes and make them your own!

Hot Infusions

A hot infusion is the classic way of making tea: you pour boiling water over herbs and let it sit. The amount of herbs to use for 1 cup of tea is quite variable. I add from 1 to 4 tablespoons per cup. If the tea tastes too strong, then you have added too much. For maximum potency, steep your herbal teas for 10 to 15 minutes. It is important to keep the tea covered while steeping, as some constituents are sensitive to heat and will evaporate.

There are all different types of tea infusers, tea bags, and teapots you can use to make tea. I use those that allow room for the leaves to "swim" around.

Cold Infusions

A cold infusion is a tea made by soaking the plant in cold water for an extended period of time. There are some plants that infuse better in cold water, usually because they have heat-sensitive compounds. Some examples of this are marshmallow root, valerian root, and fir tips. Nettle also makes a great cold infusion, though it's well suited to a hot infusion as well.

To make a cold infusion, take a quart jar and add 2 to 4 tablespoons of herbs. Fill the rest up with water, put the lid on, and put it in the fridge. Leave it for 6 to 12 hours and strain. Drink within 3 days, storing in the fridge.

Decoctions

A decoction is a tea that is boiled on the stove for a period of time. Decoctions are typically made with barks, berries, roots, and mushrooms—things that do not readily give up their constituents.

To make a typical decoction, use about 1 teaspoon of herbs per 1 cup of water. Put all of it in a pot, cover, turn the heat to medium, and bring it to a boil. Once boiling, reduce the heat and simmer for 10 minutes. I always set a timer because I tend to forget about it otherwise. Mushrooms, especially reishi and other shelf mushrooms, are typically boiled for longer periods of time. I boil them for 40 to 60 minutes.

Infusion Dosage
Dosage always depends on the herb, the person, and what you are using it for. If you are dealing with an acute condition, like a cold, you may drink 2 to 5 cups of tea a day. If you are dealing with a chronic condition, you might drink 1 cup a day.

Other Applications for Infusions
Water extracts of all types have many applications in herbalism, many of which are topical. For a compress, dip a towel in tea and apply it to an area. You can also pour tea in a bath or soak body parts in tea. Strong infusions and strong decoctions can be used to make syrups or be applied topically where oils may be too stifling.

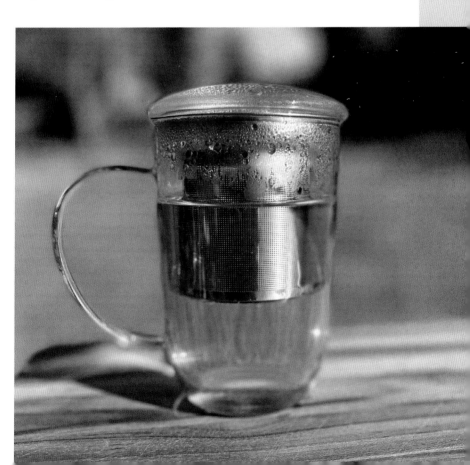

Other Preparations

There are so many ways to prepare herbs to make medicines. Some of the preparations listed here are aimed at making the medicines more palatable, some are intended to extract certain constituents, and some are made for particular applications. These are the ones I use most commonly, but of course there are many more! You will find recipes for these peppered throughout the book.

Glycerite

A glycerite is much like a tincture, with vegetable glycerin used in place of alcohol. As a solvent, vegetable glycerin is not as strong as alcohol, which means that glycerites are suitable only for certain plants. While glycerites are something I only rarely use, they are a great option for folks who prefer not to consume alcohol.

Oxymel

Oxymels have been around since the ancient Greeks. *Oxy* means "acid," and *mel* means "honey." These are a combination of vinegar and honey, often infused with herbs, and are made exactly like a tincture. They were originally used for respiratory complaints because of the anti-inflammatory and antimicrobial properties of vinegar and honey. I use a 1:1 ratio of honey to vinegar (in other words, for every 1 cup of honey, I mix in 1 cup of vinegar). See the Blackberry Oxymel and Spruce Tip Oxymel recipes.

Elixir

An elixir is much like a tincture, except some of the alcohol has been replaced with honey, which makes the medicine taste better. Honey also has its own healing properties, making elixirs especially great for sore throats, coughs, and allergies.

Cordial

A cordial has many different formulas. I use a 1:1:1 ratio: 1 part water, 1 part sugar or honey, and 1 part alcohol (40 percent or higher). You can add any amount of plant material to create the desired taste and strength. This is different from a tincture, which you want as strong and consistent as possible. A cordial can be adjusted so the flavor isn't overpowering. Cordials are a bit less alcoholic than elixirs or tinctures and can be sipped from a glass. Hawthorn berry cordial is a favorite holiday drink of mine, made with cinnamon, apples, pomegranate juice, and other spices.

Infused Honey

An herbal-infused honey is made by infusing the fresh or dry plant material in honey using a hot water bath. The honey takes on the flavor and medicinal actions of the plant. These honeys are a delicious addition to tea or as a topping for pancakes or desserts. They can also be taken by the teaspoonful for sore throats. Give more delicate plant parts, like rose petals, less time in the hot water bath, and less delicate parts, like roots and pine needles, more time. See the recipe for Rose Infused Honey.

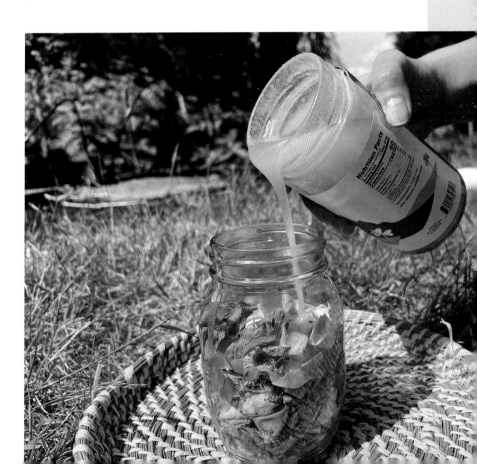

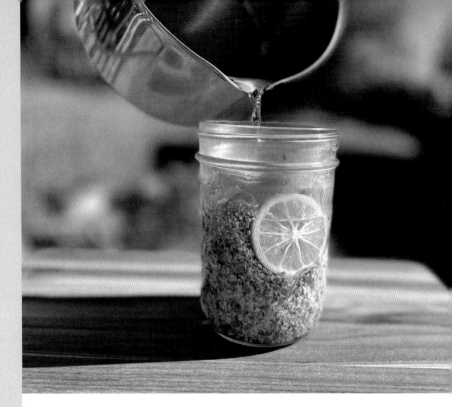

Herbal Syrup

Herbal syrups use herbs, water, and either sugar or honey. The herbs are extracted through different methods and then strained out. Homemade syrups should be kept in the refrigerator and thrown out once they show any signs of mold or bacterial growth. To see the two methods of making syrups, see the recipes for Elderflower Syrup and Blue Elderberry Syrup.

Infused Vinegar

Vinegar is great for extracting minerals and flavonoids. Make an infused vinegar like you would a folk tincture, and be sure to use a non-metal lid to avoid corrosion. Some of my favorite herbs to infuse in vinegars are fir tips, hawthorn berries, horsetail, and nettle. See the Douglas-Fir Infused Vinegar recipe.

Herbal Salt and Sugar

Herbs can also be added or infused into salts and sugars. These are usually more for nutrition and flavor than for healing in the body. See the Nettle Seed Salt recipe.

Hydrosol

A hydrosol is simply aromatic plant steam in liquid form. It is made using a still that boils the plant in water and then traps and condenses the steam. Aromatic plants are the most typical to use, like rose, mugwort, sage, rosemary, lemon balm, fir, and cedar. See the Wild Carrot Hydrosol recipe to learn how to make a crude still using common kitchen items.

Infused Oil

Infused oils are made by soaking a plant (usually wilted first) in oil for a period of time. Sometimes these are prepared with a hot water bath, and sometimes they are made just by letting them sit. To make these, wilt the herb for 24 hours (simply leave it out in the open air until it becomes limp), put it in a jar with oil, put the jar in a hot water bath in an electric slow cooker, and let it sit for 48 hours. See the recipe for Cottonwood Bud Infused Oil.

Alcohol Intermediary Oil

An alcohol intermediary oil is a type of infused oil that I have become fond of in recent years. It uses alcohol as a primary solvent, and then oil, and then the alcohol is removed through evaporation. The process is a bit more technical than the traditional method, but it makes beautiful oils. See the recipe for Bleeding Heart Alcohol Intermediary Oil.

Salve

A salve is a hardened ointment that is used topically. It is made with oil (which is usually infused with herbs first) and beeswax. Use a ratio of 1 ounce of beeswax to 7 fluid ounces of oil. You can also add essential oils to it, which 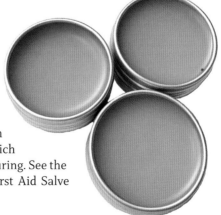 should be done right before pouring. See the recipes for Poplar and Pine First Aid Salve and Pine Resin Salve.

Storage and Shelf Life

All herbal preparations should be stored away from light and in a place that has a stable temperature. Storing preparations in amber bottles can also help block some light. Plastic lids are less likely to corrode than metal lids, so I recommend investing in some; plastic lids are essential for any acidic preparation, such as an oxymel or infused vinegar.

Tinctures have the longest shelf life of any herbal preparation and can often be stored for five years or more without losing their potency. There are certain plant tinctures that spoil or degrade more quickly and thus should be kept for only one or two years. Examples of these are nettle seed, valerian, and chickweed tinctures.

Vinegars, cordials, elixirs, and glycerites have a fairly long shelf life as well, ranging from three to five years.

Oxymels, infused honeys, and infused oils and salves have shorter shelf lives of one to three years. I often keep these preparations in the fridge to extend their shelf life. Oils are prone to

Look for small sticky paper labels at a craft store or office supply store.

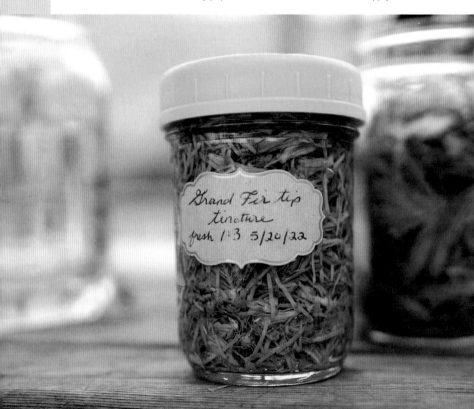

rancidity and mold easily if they were made with fresh plant material. Smell and inspect for freshness before using. Syrups must be kept in the fridge and can go bad in as quickly as one month. Adding a splash of alcohol can increase the shelf life by a few months but does not make it shelf stable.

Labels

Labeling is important to inform your future self—who will have no recollection of having made this mysterious dark liquid in the back of the cupboard—what is happening in the jar. Label everything you make with as much information as you can. Herbal medicines should be labeled with:

- the plant name
- the date the item was prepared
- alcohol percentage/menstruum information
- the ratio used
- where you harvested the plant material
- whether you used fresh or dried plant material
- medicinal uses (this is especially useful for beginners)

Part Two

The Plants and Recipes

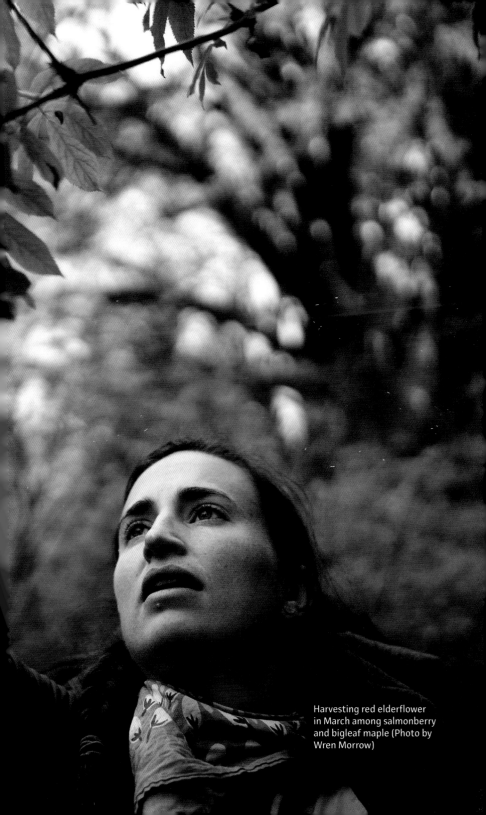

Harvesting red elderflower in March among salmonberry and bigleaf maple (Photo by Wren Morrow)

This section of the book features thirty-five local medicinal plant species, including photos, where to find them, look-alikes, how to harvest them, how to use them medicinally, and how to prepare them. Each entry has at least one basic recipe and suggestions for other preparations. Some entries will include multiple closely related species, such as in the Pine entry, with information about how to tell them apart.

Look for the skull and crossbones 💀 to indicate toxic or poisonous plants, and look for the exclamation point ❗ for look-alikes. Note that there are look-alikes that are not listed in the book, so please consult an expert if in doubt.

Recommended Materials, Ingredients, and Equipment

To make the recipes, you will need to have certain materials, ingredients, and equipment on hand. In addition to the plant material you harvest to prepare a given recipe, here are some of the most common ingredients needed for herbal medicine making:

- Apple cider vinegar
- Beeswax pastilles
- Everclear (190 proof; 95 percent)
- Granulated cane sugar
- Honey
- Organic extra-virgin olive oil
- Store-bought dried herbs and tinctures from plants not included in this book
- Vegetable glycerin
- Vodka or other 100-proof (50 percent) alcohol

The following is a list of equipment you'll likely want to have on hand:

Amber bottles. These are for dispensing or applying your medicinal preparations. I typically have 1-ounce, 2-ounce, and 4-ounce bottles on hand with spray tops (for applying tinctures topically), dropper tops (good for dosing tincture internally), and some regular screw-on tops (for long-term storage).

Blender. This is for blending herbs with liquids like oil or alcohol. Use a glass blender as the plastic ones get clouded from the alcohol and can soak up some of the intense flavors from the herbs.

Cheesecloth. This is for straining herbs out of tinctures and other preparations. I get the unbleached kind. You can also use a nut-milk bag or a piece of clean muslin fabric for this. In some cases, you'll use the cheesecloth alone, or you may use it in combination with a fine-mesh strainer.

Digital kitchen scale. Many herbal preparations use weight measurements to increase accuracy in the recipe. Get one that can display both ounces and grams.

Fine-mesh strainers. These are for straining plant material from liquids like oil and alcohol. I have small and large ones.

Food mill. This is for straining out larger seeds or pits when making jams. A food mill is not essential for medicine making, but it is useful in the chutney and jelly recipes in this book.

Food processor. A food processor is useful for making things like chickweed pesto or for chopping dandelion roots for roasting. It is not totally necessary for medicine making, but it is a nice addition to the medicine maker's kitchen.

Glass jars. Glass jars are necessary for storing both your liquid herbal preparations and dried herbs. For the recipes in this book, you'll need 8-ounce, 16-ounce, and 32-ounce jars. I prefer wide-mouth mason jars. Purchase plastic lids separately; these are critical for any preparation that is acidic as acids can corrode the standard metal lids. If left long enough, acids can actually completely eat through a metal lid!

Glass measuring cups. These are essential for accurately measuring liquids. I have a 2-ounce measuring cup, an 8-ounce measuring glass made for bartending, and a 32-ounce measuring jug with a handle.

Herb grinder. Also known as a nut-and-spice grinder, this is a small appliance used to grind up herbs into coarse powders. Cuisinart and Secura brands both make good herb grinders.

Kitchen thermometer. You will need one for measuring the temperature of certain preparations to avoid overheating them.

Small tins or jars. These are for storing salves and ointments. They come in metal, plastic, and glass. I like to use 0.5-ounce or 1-ounce tins, as they are ideal for portability and for giving as gifts.

Look to the Resources section at the back of the book for suggestions on where you can purchase some of the more specialized items.

Black Cottonwood

Populus trichocarpa
Salicaceae (willow family)

Black cottonwood trees love growing near fresh water and can usually be found on river floodplains and around lakes all over the Pacific Northwest. Because they spend their days happily sucking up groundwater, they grow very fast and tall. This fast growth means their wood is rather weak, so they are notorious for blowing over and dropping branches during windstorms.

Black cottonwood buds are filled with a sticky orange resin that drips out of the buds. This orange resin is one of the things that bees harvest and use to make propolis. Bees use propolis to seal their hives and protect the colony from infection. Propolis can be different colors, but the propolis in our area is usually orange because of the abundance of black cottonwood trees.

You will hear black cottonwood trees also referred to as poplar trees. They are in the genus *Populus*, along with aspen. Many other species of poplar have resinous buds that are used for medicine.

LEFT Harvest the leaf buds, which are filled with orange resin, for medicine. **RIGHT** If the base of the bud is black or brown, the bud is rotten and unsuitable for harvest.

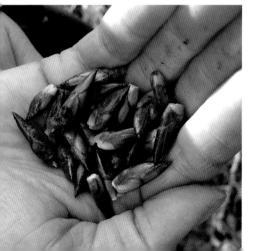
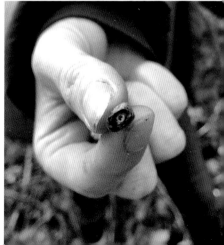

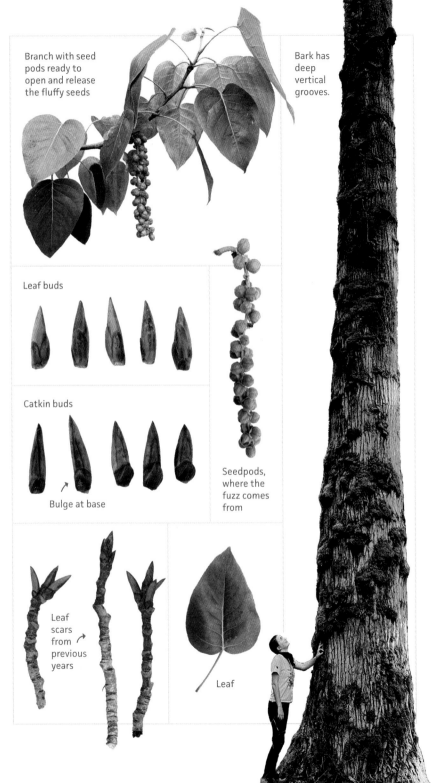

Branch with seed pods ready to open and release the fluffy seeds

Bark has deep vertical grooves.

Leaf buds

Catkin buds

Bulge at base

Seedpods, where the fuzz comes from

Leaf scars from previous years

Leaf

Harvesting Black Cottonwood

The resin-filled buds of black cottonwood can be harvested from fallen branches, or even from an entire fallen tree. Harvesting only from the nonliving tree parts makes this a lower-impact harvest. Harvest the buds in the winter months, when there are no leaves on the tree; the harvest window ends when the leaves burst out of the buds in spring. Because the resin is an important part of the medicine, aim for harvesting in January and February, when there is the most resin.

There are two main types of buds: catkin buds and leaf buds. Only the leaf buds have a good amount of resin in them, so I harvest those. The leaf buds are most often at the tip of each branch and sometimes on the branches' sides. To distinguish between the two types of buds, squeeze them. The leaf buds will be squishy, and the catkin buds will be dry and hard. You can also pull a bud apart to see whether it has tiny leaves (leaf buds) or a corn-like structure inside (catkin buds).

COTTONWOOD BUD THROAT SPRAY   *Makes 2 ounces*

For this recipe, you'll need to have four different tinctures on hand, plus honey. You can prepare your own black cottonwood bud tincture (see Tincture Ratio Chart) and purchase the others, or purchase all four. Use this spray for a sore throat preceding a cold or flu, or for a sore throat of bacterial origin.

Dosage: Spray onto the back of the throat 2 to 10 times a day, depending on severity.

---

1 tablespoon black cottonwood bud tincture
  (see Tincture Ratio Chart)
1 tablespoon echinacea root tincture
1 tablespoon sage leaf tincture
1½ teaspoons licorice root tincture
1½ teaspoons honey

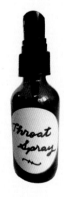

Combine all the ingredients in a 2-ounce amber spray bottle, screw on the top, and shake gently to mix.

Make sure the honey is thoroughly dissolved to prevent clogging the sprayer.

The throat spray will keep for 3 years. Over time, gloppy precipitates may form that clog the sprayer. You can strain the mixture through a piece of cheesecloth if this happens.

If the branch has been on the ground for a month or two, the buds can be rotten inside, so check the broken base of the bud after picking to see if there are streaks of brown or black (see photo on page 56). If it's greenish white, you're good!

Harvest buds into a parchment-paper bag or directly into the jar in which you will make your medicine. The resin will stick to paper and plastic and will definitely ruin fabric.

POPLAR AND PINE FIRST AID SALVE
Makes eight 0.5-ounce tins

Use this salve as a topical antimicrobial for cuts (like cat scratches), or just because it smells good. It can also be good for joint pain of cold origin; a stiff joint helped by heat may fall into that category. Harvest your own pine resin (see the Douglas-Fir, Fir, Pine, and Spruce entries for instructions) or purchase resin online (see Resources). Be sure to weigh and measure the ingredients carefully; measuring matters for the consistency of the salve. For the salve jars, I use small metal tins.

Dosage: Rub a small amount of salve on a healing cut or sore joint 2 times a day.

3.5 fluid ounces Cottonwood Bud Infused
    Oil (see next recipe)
0.8 ounce pine resin
0.5 ounce beeswax pastilles

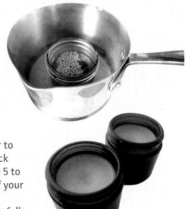

Add the oil, resin, and beeswax to an old, clean 16-ounce jar. The jar is very hard to clean, so I often end up tossing it out after using it.

Place the jar, uncovered, in a medium saucepan. Add enough water to the pan to reach the level of oil in the jar. Put the pan on medium heat, bring the water to a simmer, and stir the mixture with a chopstick until everything is dissolved. This should take 5 to 10 minutes. During this time, take the lids off your salve tins and line them up on a paper towel.

Once all the ingredients have liquefied, carefully remove the jar and pour the mixture into the waiting tins. Leave the tins open on a level surface until they harden completely.

Label and store the tins for 1 to 5 years. Check for rancidity by smell—rancid oils smell sour and pungent in an unpleasant way. Because poplar bud and pine resin are preservatives, this salve doesn't go rancid as quickly as other oils.

Medicinal Uses of Black Cottonwood

An important part of the medicinal action of cottonwood buds lies in their sticky orange resin. Plants use resin to prevent and treat infections. For example, pine trees create resin to fill holes in the bark, protecting the tree much like a scab does for our wounds. Without this resin, fungus and insects can enter these holes and cause disease on the inner part of the tree, which can be fatal. Black cottonwood buds create resin to prevent the baby leaves inside the bud from rotting in the cold,

COTTONWOOD BUD INFUSED OIL *Makes 8 ounces*

This aromatic infused oil can be used as an antimicrobial salve, for pain relief, to stimulate circulation, or as a massage oil. If the buds were wet when harvesting, lay them out on parchment paper to dry for 24 hours first.

Dosage: Rub the oil into hands, wrists, knees, and neck as needed, or use it as a massage oil.

1 cup fresh cottonwood buds
1 cup organic extra-virgin olive oil, plus
   more as needed

Add the cottonwood buds to a clean 16-ounce jar and pour the oil over the buds until they are covered.

Add a couple of inches of water to the bottom of a slow cooker and set the jar of oil and buds inside, uncovered. Adjust the water level to ensure it meets the level of oil in the jar. Avoid getting water in the jar at any point in the process. Set the slow cooker to warm (low works but sometimes can get a bit too hot), and leave the lid off.

Let the jar sit in the slow cooker for 12 to 48 hours. The longer it sits, the stronger the oil will be. Monitor periodically and add more water as the water line drops.

If you do not have a slow cooker, you can make a hot water bath with a couple of inches of water in a medium saucepan on a stove set to the lowest heat, but you will need to watch it more attentively and turn it off overnight. Don't let the water boil!

You will know the oil is ready when it smells fragrant. It may fill your whole house with the smell of cottonwood buds.

Strain the oil with a fine-mesh strainer into a clean, dry 8-ounce jar and put the lid on. Store the oil in the fridge. It will keep for 1 to 3 years.

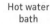
Hot water bath

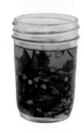
Leave the lid off when heating.

wet winter. If you pull apart a cottonwood bud, you will find the tiny leaves happily encased in the resin. You can spread this resin directly on a scratch or cut to prevent infection. More commonly, herbalists infuse the buds in oil to make an antimicrobial salve (see Cottonwood Bud Infused Oil and Poplar and Pine First Aid Salve). Oil infused with black cottonwood buds is also used to relieve pain as it is anti-inflammatory and stimulates circulation.

Like other aromatic and resinous herbs (such as pine resin, white sage, and gumweed), black cottonwood buds are antimicrobial and expectorant, making them very suitable for wet coughs, lung infections, and throat infections. I add black cottonwood bud tincture to throat sprays (see Cottonwood Bud Throat Spray) or infuse the buds in honey and stir a teaspoon into a cup of thyme tea for a stubborn, phlegmy cough.

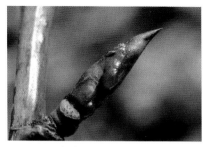

Orange resin leaks out of a cottonwood bud on a warm winter day.

The bark of most of the members of the willow family contains salicylic acid, an anti-inflammatory compound that can help with pain relief, much like aspirin. Black cottonwood doesn't taste great, so I tend not to use it internally like I would willow bark (see the Willow entry). However, the bark of quaking aspen (*Populus tremuloides*), a close relative of black cottonwood, is more tasty and is used as a tincture and tea for its pain-relieving qualities.

Making Medicine with Black Cottonwood

The parts of black cottonwood most frequently used in medicine are the buds. Because of their high resin content, the best solvents to extract the medicinal constituents are high-proof alcohol and oil.

In addition to the infused oil and salve recipes included here, you can make a tincture of the fresh buds with very high-proof alcohol (see Tincture Ratio Chart), which is used in the Cottonwood Bud Throat Spray recipe. You can also make a strong infused honey with the fresh buds (see the Rose Infused Honey recipe for instructions on how to make an infused honey).

Blackberry

Rubus ursinus, R. bifrons
Rosaceae (rose family)

Three species of blackberry grow widely in the Pacific Northwest: the native trailing blackberry (*Rubus ursinus*), the aggressively invasive Himalayan blackberry (*Rubus bifrons*), and the less common laceleaf blackberry (*Rubus laciniatus;* not covered here).

Did you know that Himalayan blackberry is a human-bred species? It was meticulously bred by botanist and horticulturist Luther Burbank in Northern California in the late nineteenth century. He was trying to create a fruit that would be thornless, prolific in the Northwest, and delicious. It took only a few years for the Himalayan blackberry (so named because the original seed was said to have come from India) to become roaringly popular—starts of it were sent all over. After that, birds continued its spread and Himalayan blackberry quickly naturalized throughout our bioregion, proving its incredible fitness. The original variety was thornless, but it quickly developed thorns again in the wild, as thornlessness is a recessive trait.

Today, Himalayan blackberry is one of the most invasive plants of our bioregion. It grows in shade and sun, and in dry and wet soil. Burbank's obsession with genetic strength really shows in this plant!

As a result of this colorful history, we have more wild blackberry available to us here than anywhere else in the world, so

LEFT Trailing blackberry in flower, with cleavers and holly in the background **RIGHT** Ripe Himalayan blackberries in abundance at a local park

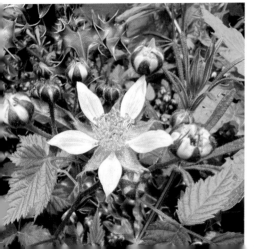
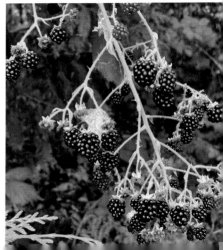

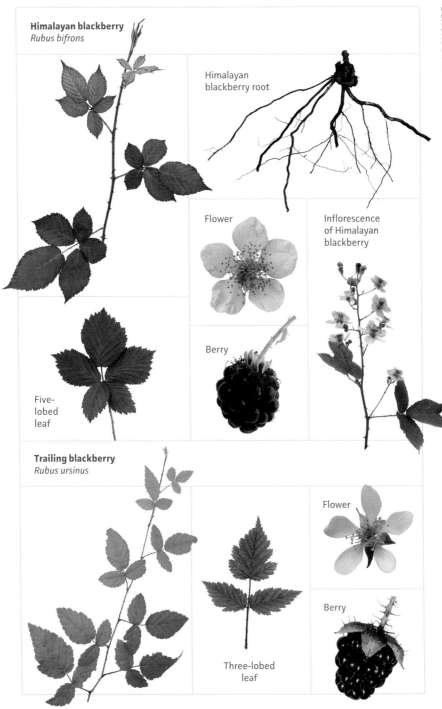

Himalayan blackberry
Rubus bifrons

Himalayan blackberry root

Flower

Inflorescence of Himalayan blackberry

Berry

Five-lobed leaf

Trailing blackberry
Rubus ursinus

Three-lobed leaf

Flower

Berry

I just had to include it in this book. All parts of the blackberry plant can be used medicinally, the berries are wonderfully edible, and baskets can even be made of the canes if processed correctly.

Blackberry leaves have historically been used for medicine across Western and Eastern Europe—especially Russia. When I worked at an herb store, I sold blackberry leaves almost exclusively to older Russian women. I asked one of them what she used it for, and she said that she used it for balancing blood sugar!

Harvesting Blackberry

The root of blackberry is hard and stubborn. It should be dug in the spring or fall, as with all other roots, but opportunistic harvests in other seasons are not to be turned down. Using a digging fork, loosen the soil around the root and then pop it out of the ground. You may need to use your hands to coax it a bit.

The leaves can be harvested when they are just emerging in April or later on in May or June. After that, they start to get dry and not as palatable. Wear gloves as all species of blackberries have thorns.

The berries of trailing blackberry ripen first in July and are, in my opinion, the best tasting of the three species. They typically grow in the forest, but the vines that get the most sunlight

LEFT Harvesting the root of a monstrous Himalayan blackberry that found its way into the forest
RIGHT To clean roots, blast them with a garden hose. Then scrub them again in the sink with a brush.

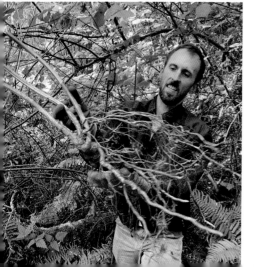
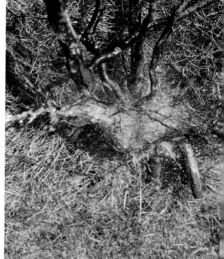

will have the most berries, so seek trailing blackberry in open fields.

Himalayan and laceleaf blackberry both ripen in August. When harvesting, wear long sleeves, gloves, and thick pants, especially for Himalayan. Watch for bees' nests, as they like to set up camp under blackberry patches.

Medicinal Uses of Blackberry

Historically, blackberry leaf tea has been used for diabetes—research confirms this use. The leaves share some similar compounds with red raspberry leaves, which means they can be used for menstrual issues and fertility, where a toning, astringent

---

BLACKBERRY ROOT TINCTURE   *Makes 5 ounces*

A tincture made from blackberry roots is useful for treating GI conditions like diarrhea and dysentery as well as for dental hygiene. The recipe includes vegetable glycerin to make some of the constituents stay in solution. If you harvest your own blackberry roots, spray them with a garden hose on the jet setting. This will get the first layer of dirt off. Then bring them inside and finish scrubbing them with a scrub brush and a bowl of water.

Dosage: Take small doses of about 10 drops as needed.

2.5 ounces fresh blackberry root, cleaned thoroughly
4.5 fluid ounces 100-proof alcohol (50 percent), such as vodka
0.5 fluid ounce vegetable glycerin

Use clippers to cut the clean root into the smallest pieces you can manage, ¼ inch or smaller.

Add the root pieces to a clean 8-ounce jar and pour the alcohol and glycerin over the root pieces. Secure the lid on the jar and let sit for 4 weeks in a cool, dark place.

After 4 weeks, strain the tincture through cheesecloth and store in an 8-ounce jar. The tincture will keep for 5 years. Dispense into a 1-ounce dropper bottle to carry and use.

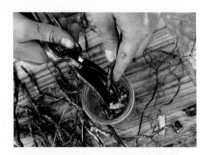
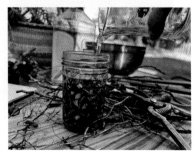

action is needed. The leaves are also fairly high in iron, as are the berries. The most common use of the leaves is as a gastrointestinal (GI) tract astringent, effectively drying out and reinforcing tissue. This could be helpful where there's infection or loss of tone in the intestines. Many rose-family plants are used for the GI tract due to their astringent and cooling compounds. Examples include rose petals, agrimony, avens, apple twigs, and raspberry leaf.

The root is the most astringent part of the blackberry plant, making it the best part to use for cases that really need that tightening and drying effect. It is used for diarrhea and dysentery especially. It can also be used for spongy gums or loose teeth as a tincture or mouthwash, or it can be chewed directly. For the tincture, start with only 10 drops, and then add another 10 if that doesn't work. I know from personal experience that it is actually pretty potent.

BLACKBERRY OXYMEL   *Makes about 1 cup*

Serve with soda water, ice, and a squeeze of lime or lemon as a refreshing sweet-and-sour beverage. Though most oxymels can be made and stored at room temperature, this particular oxymel gains water from the berries, making it less shelf stable, and thus should be kept in the fridge as a precaution.

½ cup honey
½ cup apple cider vinegar
1½ cups blackberries, fresh or frozen

In a 4-cup measuring jug, combine the honey and vinegar and stir until the honey is dissolved.

Put the berries in a clean 16-ounce jar and pour the vinegar and honey mixture over them. Let sit in the refrigerator for 1 week.

Strain through cheesecloth, squeezing the juice out of the berries, and transfer the oxymel to another 16-ounce jar with a plastic lid. Store in the fridge for up to 1 year.

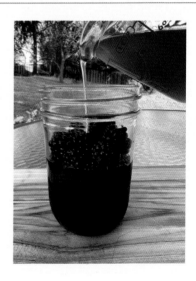

The berries are high in iron, vitamin C, and various antioxidants. In Chinese medicine, blackberries are thought to tonify the kidneys, like other purple and black foods.

Making Medicine with Blackberry

There are only two medicinal preparations I recommend for this plant: a hot infusion of the dried leaf and a tincture of the fresh or dried root (see Tincture Ratio Chart).

All kinds of edible delights can be made with the berry, which is beyond the scope of this book. However, I did include a very nice Blackberry Oxymel recipe, which is a classic herbal preparation made with vinegar and honey. Oxymels were originally used as respiratory medicine by the ancient Greeks. Nowadays they are often used to make a refreshing summer beverage (see recipe).

Cautions

Blackberry root is very drying and can cause constipation if taken when not needed or in too large a dose.

Bleeding Heart

Dicentra formosa
Papaveraceae (poppy family)

Pacific bleeding heart (*Dicentra formosa*) is a surprisingly abundant native plant of forest understories. When using this plant for medicine, keep in mind that Pacific bleeding heart is a toxic plant, which makes dosage very important (see Cautions).

The abundance of bleeding heart in Pacific Northwest forests west of the Cascades is likely attributable to the fact that it can thrive in a variety of conditions: it doesn't require old growth or anything like that; it will take second and third growth, and even make its way up among English ivy if there's room. You can transplant it into a shady, mulched area of your garden and it will spread readily. It has delicate leaves with a bluish hue that catch dewdrops beautifully.

There are other cultivated varieties of bleeding heart that are popular in gardens throughout the region. These theoretically have the same medicinal properties, though little information is available about their medicinal uses.

Harvesting Bleeding Heart

Pacific bleeding heart tends to flower in April but can flower into June high in the mountains. Try to select a robust and thick patch of Pacific bleeding heart to harvest from. Thin out the patch in some of the thick spots, and the hole you made should

LEFT Bleeding heart in full flower **RIGHT** A bleeding heart leaf emerging from a bed of alder leaves in early spring

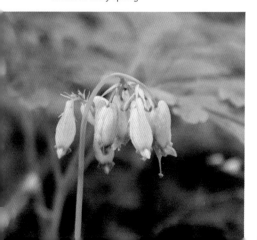
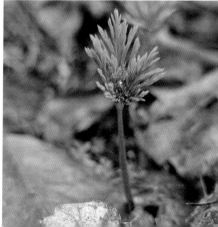

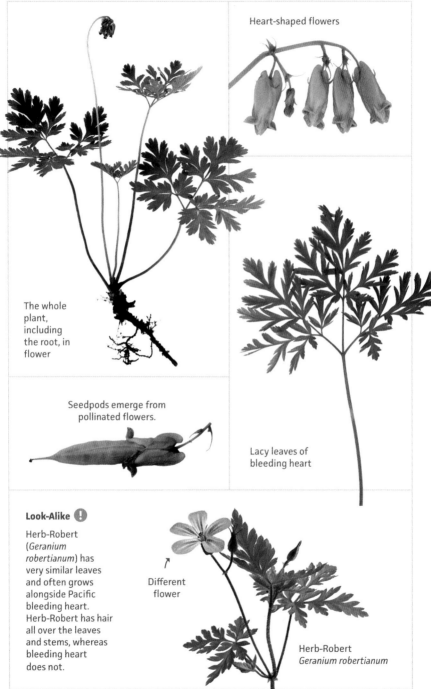

Heart-shaped flowers

The whole plant, including the root, in flower

Seedpods emerge from pollinated flowers.

Lacy leaves of bleeding heart

Look-Alike ⚠️

Herb-Robert (*Geranium robertianum*) has very similar leaves and often grows alongside Pacific bleeding heart. Herb-Robert has hair all over the leaves and stems, whereas bleeding heart does not.

Different flower

Herb-Robert
Geranium robertianum

fill back in quickly. You can also aid the patch by pulling out English ivy if you find it creeping nearby.

Bleeding heart spreads by underground rhizomes, so to harvest, tug gently to remove the roots that run parallel to the ground under the leaf duff. The roots are the most potent part of the plant, so be sure to get as much out of the ground as you can. Some herbalists might use only the root, but it takes a lot to amount to anything useful because the roots are so thin, and I don't like to waste the flowering tops. I use the whole plant in flower, which means the roots, leaves, stems, and flowers.

Medicinal Uses of Bleeding Heart

Bleeding heart is primarily a central-nervous-system sedative and is used for relieving pain topically and internally. I use bleeding heart for menstrual cramps, migraine headaches, and tooth pain. It can also be a great ally for moments of extreme anxiety or shock. In fact, bleeding heart tincture would be a great addition to a first aid kit. The alcohol intermediary oil of this plant (see recipe) can be used topically for menstrual pain, back pain, neck pain, and joint pain in general.

It is hard to find written information on using any species of bleeding heart, such as drug interactions and contraindications. This is interesting, because most herbalists in our bioregion that I have talked to use it often. This is a great example of a case where bioregional folk traditions still exist but are too localized to reach academia.

LEFT Carefully pulling out bleeding heart rhizomes by hand **RIGHT** Bleeding heart rhizomes run in mats parallel to the ground. They are thin and delicate, and are easiest to harvest from soft leaf duff.

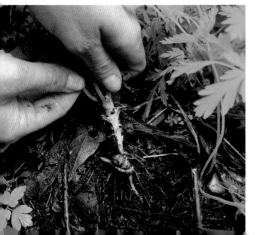
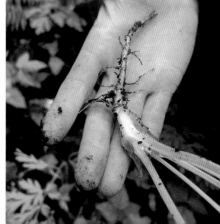

BLEEDING HEART ALCOHOL INTERMEDIARY OIL   *Makes 8 to 10 ounces*

This pain-relieving oil can be applied topically to sore joints for mild pain relief.

Dosage: Rub oil onto affected area several times a day.

2 ounces dried bleeding heart (whole
   plant), cut into small pieces
1.5 fluid ounces 190-proof alcohol
   (95 percent), such as Everclear
10 fluid ounces organic extra-virgin olive oil

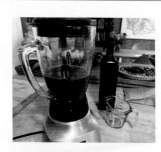

Grind the bleeding heart pieces in an herb grinder until they reach the consistency of coarse sand.

Put the ground plant material into a clean 16-ounce jar and add the alcohol. Mix with a fork until the plant material is evenly coated. Seal the jar with the lid and let sit at room temperature for 2 to 24 hours. The longer you let it sit, the better your extraction will be.

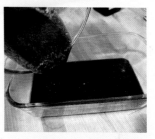

Preheat the oven to 170°F (this is the "warm" setting on my oven). Pour the contents of the jar into a blender. Add the oil and blend on medium-low for 5 minutes until thoroughly blended. The resulting green mixture should have the consistency of a smoothie and pour easily.

Pour the mixture into a 9-by-9-inch glass baking dish and warm in the oven for 2 to 3 hours. The goal here is to extract more by using a bit of heat before you strain the oil.

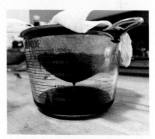

Strain the oil through a fine-mesh strainer lined with a piece of cheesecloth.

After straining, let the alcohol evaporate. Alcohol is lighter than oil, so it will naturally separate out and float to the top. It evaporates easily, even at room temperature. Cover the container loosely with fabric and let it sit for a few days. To speed up the process, just pop it back into the warm oven and it will be done in just an hour or two. You will know there is no more alcohol when the smell of alcohol goes away.

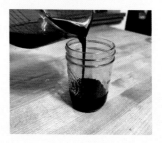

Pour the oil into a clean, dry 8- or 16-ounce jar (depending on yield) and store in the refrigerator for 2 to 3 years. Label it well!

Making Medicine with Bleeding Heart

When working with low-dose plants internally, a standardized tincture is the preferred preparation over a folk tincture as the standardized method makes it is easier to take consistent and predictable doses. Anytime you change the concentration of a tincture, the dosage will be different. For nontoxic plants, consistency is less of a concern, but for toxic plants like bleeding heart, always make consistent medicine so that your dosage does not drastically change from batch to batch (see Tincture Ratio Chart). For internal use, I take from 5 to 20 drops of bleeding heart tincture.

Another preparation I make is Bleeding Heart Alcohol Intermediary Oil (see recipe). This involves drying the plant, grinding it up, and mixing it with a bit of alcohol before blending it with oil. The alcohol step is necessary for bleeding heart because of the alcohol-soluble nature of some of the constituents. The result is a deep-green pain-relieving oil that can be used topically. I have seen it relieve back pain within minutes. You could even combine it half and half with cannabis oil or CBD oil to increase the action.

Cautions

Bleeding heart is toxic when used internally, as mentioned. For internal use, do not exceed 20 drops of the tincture in one dose, and stop taking immediately if any undesirable symptoms come up. Toxic symptoms include extreme sedation, breathing difficulty, nausea, vomiting, and diarrhea. This herb is not safe for pregnant women, children, or animals. Also, do not take this herb internally with any pharmaceutical sedative. Because this is a lesser-known and lesser-used plant, not much is known about the herb-and-drug interactions, so it's best to be cautious.

California Poppy

Eschscholzia californica
Papaveraceae (poppy family)

This poppy, native to California and Oregon, loves to grow in rocky slopes, sidewalk cracks, and grassy hillsides. In Washington, I see it naturalized most often in gardens, and occasionally in the wild. Once it is established in your garden, it will eagerly reseed itself if you let it.

California poppy is part of a handful of plants in the poppy family that grow wild in our area, along with bleeding heart (*Dicentra formosa*). Most of these plants are valuable medicines due to their action on the central nervous system.

Harvesting California Poppy

Harvest either the aerial parts in flower (everything aboveground) or the whole plant in flower (including the root) in May through September. I typically harvest in June from my yard, where there is a wild population that has established itself. Use scissors to snip off the aboveground parts, or get a small trowel to unearth the whole plant.

The roots leak a striking bright-orange sap when cut and can be harvested for separate use. I avoid digging them up by the roots in the wild, but I do dig them up in gardens, where they easily reseed and can become weedy.

LEFT One of my students harvesting California poppy in flower **RIGHT** A California poppy flower unfurling in a local community garden (Photo by Wren Morrow)

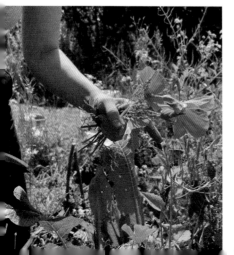 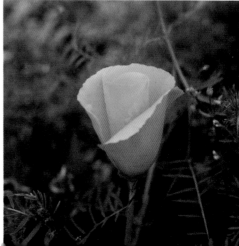

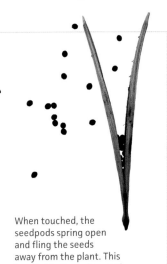

When touched, the seedpods spring open and fling the seeds away from the plant. This is called ballistic dispersal.

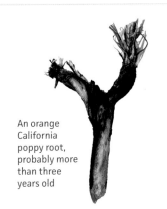

An orange California poppy root, probably more than three years old

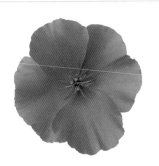

Flowers have four petals and bright-orange pollen

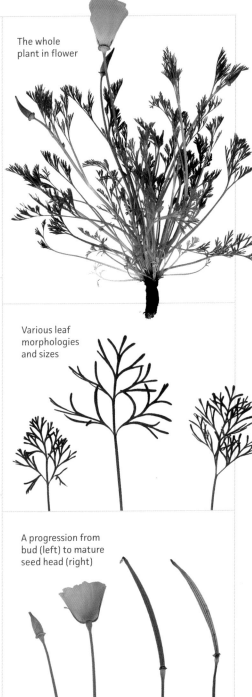

The whole plant in flower

Various leaf morphologies and sizes

A progression from bud (left) to mature seed head (right)

Medicinal Uses of California Poppy

California poppy is quite safe, even suitable for use with children. It is sedative and analgesic (pain relieving), making it good for sleep, pain, and anxiety.

California poppy is the herb I use most often to help me fall asleep. I take 1 dropperful of the tincture about an hour before going to bed, and then another dropperful right as I am turning out the lights. Note that most people feel drowsy the morning after taking this.

California poppy is often combined with other sedative herbs for sleep formulas, most notably valerian root. To do this, you can make a tincture combining them together in equal parts—an ounce of each in a 2-ounce bottle.

Try using California poppy tincture internally for pain associated with headaches (especially those with an anxiety component), menstrual cramps, and tooth pain.

Dosing Herbs for Pain

There are several dosing strategies to consider when working with acute pain. For migraines, it can be helpful to take doses of the herb every hour or so. Start with 30 drops (1 dropperful) of the tincture per hour. You can also front-load a dose, which means that the initial dose is larger. So you might take 60 drops the first dose, then take 30 drops an hour later, and 30 drops again an hour after that. One other strategy is to crowd the initial few doses, which means you might take the second dose only 15 minutes after the first, then the next one 30 minutes after that, then gaps of 1 hour after that. When using frequent doses like this, it is important to pay attention to how you feel as some herbs can have negative side effects if taken in large amounts.

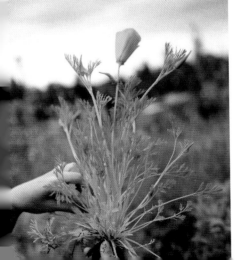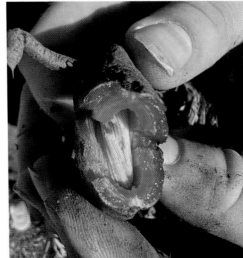

LEFT Harvesting the whole plant in flower (Photo by Wren Morrow) RIGHT The roots of California poppy have bright-orange sap inside.

Research shows it to be effective for reducing anxiety. To use it for this effect, you could combine it with other herbs like lemon balm.

As with other sedative herbs, you will build up a tolerance to the sedative powers of California poppy the more you use it, and you may find yourself needing larger doses as time goes on. Your body learns how to clear it more efficiently each time, much like it would a toxin. I take periodic breaks from sedative herbs, sometimes monthslong, which serves to resensitize my system to them.

Making Medicine with California Poppy

California poppy does not taste great, which means that making tea with it is not the best option. Instead, I use the tincture (see Fresh California Poppy Tincture). Start with a dose of 1 dropperful (about 30 drops) for an adult. Keep in mind that dosages for children are much lower, depending on their size and age. Refer to the book *Herbs for Children's Health* by Rosemary Gladstar for more information about using herbs for children.

Some herbalists claim to use the root topically for pain because it is more potent than the aerial parts. An acrid flavor tends to

SLEEP BLEND   *Makes 2 ounces*

Sometimes sedative herbs work better together. Rather than taking just one herb for sleep, I like to make formulas with two or three herbs in them. Note that you may feel groggy in the morning after taking this for-mula. The sedative actions of these herbs make this blend useful for pain as well.

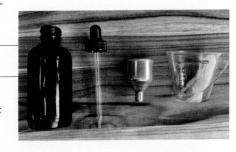

Dosage: Take 30 to 60 drops before bed.

4 teaspoons Fresh California Poppy
   Tincture (see recipe), or store-bought
4 teaspoons lemon balm tincture
4 teaspoons valerian root tincture

Combine the tinctures in a 2-ounce amber dropper bottle, and store upright in a cool, dry place.

This tincture will keep for up to 1 year; after that, the effect of grogginess will worsen as the valerian tincture ages.

be a sign of pain-relieving or antispasmodic qualities in a plant, and raw California poppy roots are acrid enough to make your tongue burn, so it makes sense that they would make a good pain reliever. The roots being more medicinally potent than the aerial parts is commonly known, and this fact also applies to other plants, such as angelica and Pacific bleeding heart.

Cautions

Do not take California poppy with pharmaceutical sedative medications. This is true of any herb with a sedative action as the combined effect can create too much sedation and inhibit breathing.

FRESH CALIFORNIA POPPY TINCTURE *Makes 10 ounces*

This tincture can be used to aid sleep, relieve pain, and reduce anxiety. You can use this tincture straight or combine it with tinctures of other herbs (see Sleep Blend). I first blend the whole fresh plant with the alcohol to increase the available surface area. If you want to make the tincture from the dried plant, you can grind the plant parts first (find the right ratio in the Tincture Ratio Chart). Note that you may feel drowsy the morning after taking this tincture.

Dosage: Take 30 to 60 drops under the tongue before bed.

2.5 ounces fresh California poppy
(whole plant in flower)
7.5 fluid ounces 190-proof alcohol
(95 percent), such as Everclear

Chop the plant parts into small pieces.
    Add the plant material and the alcohol to a blender and blend until it is a chunky pulp, 1 to 2 minutes. You may need to stir it a few times as it will be thick.
    Pour the mixture into a clean 16-ounce jar, close the lid tightly, and label well. Let sit for 4 weeks in a cool, dark place.
    Strain the mixture through a fine-mesh strainer and pour it back into the 16-ounce jar you made it in. Store it away from heat and light and dispense into smaller dropper bottles as needed. The tincture will keep for up to 5 years.

Cedar

Thuja plicata, Callitropsis nootkatensis
Cupressaceae (cypress family)

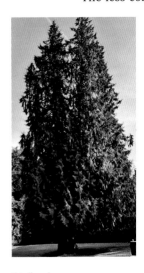

We have two native species of cedar in Washington, and they are actually not in the same genus and not considered true cedars. The less common Alaska yellow cedar (*Callitropsis nootkatensis*) grows in the mountains and is not featured in this book. The most common species is, of course, western redcedar (*Thuja plicata*). Western redcedar is a common tree in the moist forests of the Pacific Northwest.

The wood of cedar is so antifungal that it takes an extra long time to decompose. That is why cedar is often a preferred building material in the Pacific Northwest, traditionally used for roofs, because other woods would rot more quickly in the wet weather.

Cedar is one of the most important trees for the Indigenous peoples of this area, who have a long tradition of processing the bark and using it to make elaborately woven garments that are soft, water repellent, and resistant to mold and mildew. Many Native people continue to make beautiful baskets and hats from cedar harvested and processed in the traditional way. The wood of cedar—because of its strength and resilience—is used to make canoes, totem poles, longhouses, water-transport containers, tools, and many other items.

A tall cedar with a split trunk

LEFT The scaled leaves of western redcedar **RIGHT** The branches of western redcedar swoop upward and the leaves droop downward.

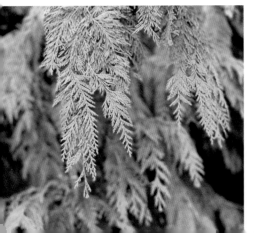

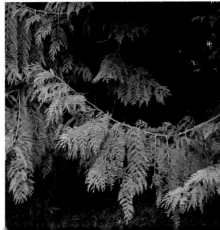

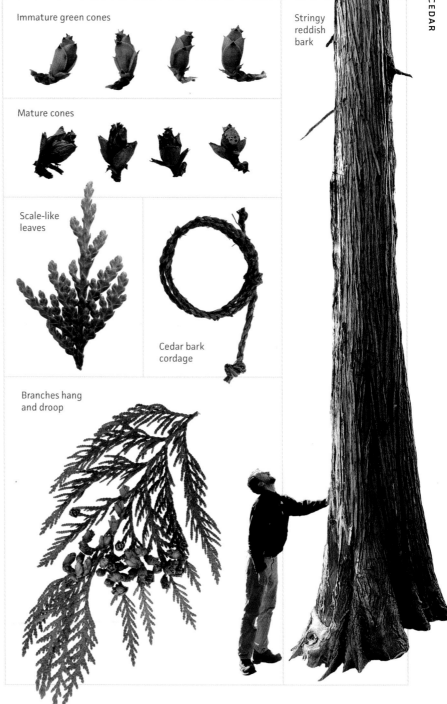

Immature green cones

Mature cones

Scale-like leaves

Cedar bark cordage

Branches hang and droop

Stringy reddish bark

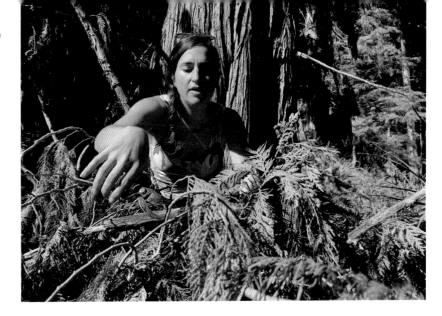

Harvest-
ing cedar
leaves from
a downed
tree. Rescue
medicinal
plants from
areas slated
for develop-
ment when
you can!

Harvesting Cedar

Harvest young, brighter-green leaves for medicine in the summer or fall. Test the leaves for aroma; they should smell strong
and lovely. The leaves rarely mold during the drying process,
but they do take a while to get completely crunchy and dry—
about 2 to 4 weeks.

I do not harvest the bark from live trees for two reasons: (1)
harvesting the bark sustainably, without killing or damaging
the tree, requires skill and knowledge, and (2) harvesting cedar
bark is a core cultural practice that does not belong to me.
However, if I come upon a recently downed tree, I will harvest
the bark and have made nice cordage from it.

Medicinal Uses of Cedar

The main uses of cedar capitalize on its strong antifungal properties. Cedar is used topically for ringworm, athlete's foot, and
any skin fungus. Either a cedar infused oil or a cedar essential oil is typically used, the latter being strong but more likely
to irritate the skin. A good compromise here is to mix some
essential oil into your infused oil to give it stronger antifungal
properties.

Cedar is also active against certain viruses. Cedar supposi-
tories and douches are used to fight human papillomavirus

CEDAR SMOKE STICKS   *Makes 1 smoke stick*

Using bundles of aromatic plants for ceremonies and rituals is an ancient tradition. In Europe, this practice was especially common in times of disease. It was believed that diseases were "vapors" that could be chased away or repelled by herbal incense and smoke. Many North American Indigenous traditions use bundles called "smudge sticks" that have ritual purposes. Look up the traditions around smoke cleansing from your own ancestral line! You can make your smoke stick small or large, depending on your preference.

Fresh cedar leaves
About 2 feet of thin hemp cord

Cut pieces of fresh cedar leaves into 5-inch lengths (or your desired length). Pile them up in a stack 1 to 2 inches high.

Start wrapping the hemp cord around one end of the stack. Wrap the cord over the tail of the thread to hold it in place, then continue wrapping toward the other end of the bundle. Wrap it tightly because the cedar leaves will shrink as they dry.

When you get to the end, wrap back to the beginning and tie off.

Leave the bundle to dry for a week or so in a place with good air flow, like a basket or a drying rack.

When ready to use, ignite a bundle with a lighter or candle. This should create an ember, which you can blow on to create more smoke. Don't overignite, as it will create too much smoke and the bundle will burn too quickly.

Extinguish in sand or with water. Never set it on a flammable surface. I use a ceramic platter for smoke sticks and incense. Note that burning a smoke stick could set off a smoke alarm.

Store unused bundles in a cool, dry place for up to 1 year. Discard when they lose their scent.

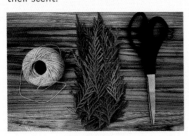 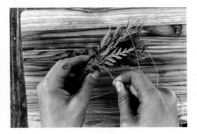

(HPV) infections, which can cause abnormal pap findings and, later, cervical cancer.

Though there are a number of traditional internal uses, including for rheumatism and coughs, I choose not to use cedar internally because of its potential toxic effect on the kidneys.

But some herbalists include a small amount of cedar in formulas for colds, flus, and bronchitis. Energetically, the smoke of cedar is believed to clear energy and is a prime candidate if you would like to cleanse space. That makes a lot of sense with the ample antimicrobial actions of this tree.

Making Medicine with Cedar

Cedar alcohol intermediary oil is delightfully green and fragrant. I make mine with freshly dried cedar leaves and olive oil. A friend of mine makes a wonderful salve that contains calendula, cedar, and poplar bud oil, which I have seen work on all kinds of rash-type skin irritations, like dermatitis, eczema, and psoriasis. To use the infused oil for a fungal infection, I add a bit of cedar essential oil (try 20 drops per ounce of oil) to strengthen the action.

An infusion of dried cedar leaves can be used as a wash, footbath, bath, or douche.

Cedar hydrosol smells lovely. It's easy to make with the abundant cedar branches that get trimmed from or fall off the tree. I use it as an antimicrobial spray on wounds.

It is also common for people to make smoke sticks (see recipe) or loose incense from cedar.

People do make cedar leaf tincture (see Tincture Ratio Chart), which can be used internally and externally. Due to concerns about toxicity (see Cautions), I don't use cedar tincture internally and prefer the oil for topical use.

Cautions

Cedar is not suitable for use during pregnancy. It can be toxic if taken internally in larger doses due to it containing thujone, a toxic compound that can cause convulsions, kidney damage, and other adverse symptoms.

Chickweed

Stellaria media
Caryophyllaceae (pink family)

Chickweed, more formally known as common chickweed (*Stellaria media*), is a very adaptable, non-native weed that grows abundantly in the Pacific Northwest. It also grows in every single state in the United States and is common in several other temperate countries.

You will find chickweed growing in disturbed areas that are moist, such as lawns, garden beds, and parks. The largest chickweed patch I have ever seen was growing in an old manure pile at the back of a forested property, presumably enjoying the soft and nutrient-dense manure. It also seems to have a penchant for finding small patches of soil in cities and taking them over when nothing else will grow.

Common chickweed has many look-alikes, so make sure to inspect it closely to get your ID right. The most common look-alike I have seen is sticky mouse-eared chickweed (*Cerastium glomeratum*), which is also edible. It's not eaten as much as common chickweed, probably because it is covered in hair and thus not as enjoyable. The *Cerastium* genus has many other members that look very similar to common chickweed as well. In Washington State, we also have several native species in the same genus as chickweed (*Stellaria*), which are less common than common chickweed.

LEFT A healthy patch of common chickweed growing in a local park **RIGHT** Notice the single line of hairs on the stem, a specific characteristic of common chickweed.

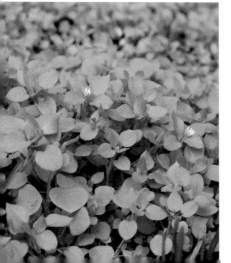
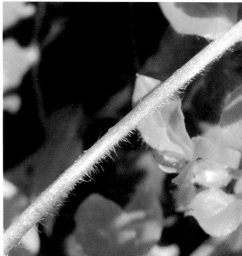

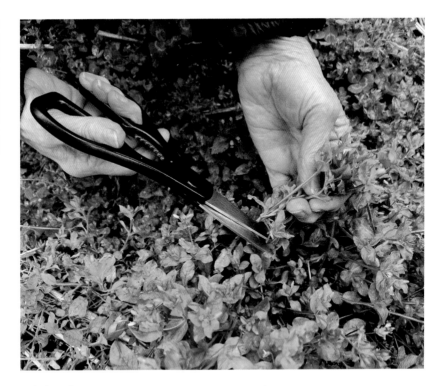

A chickweed harvest is a lot like giving a haircut. Use scissors to snip off the leafy ends.

Harvesting Chickweed

Harvest chickweed tops in early spring before the plant flowers for the most delicious, tender plant material. Use scissors to trim the nice green leaves off the top, leaving the roots and lower leaves so it might sprout again. The stems will become more and more fibrous the older the plant gets and the longer it is in bloom. It's still edible when fibrous, but it becomes much less pleasant to eat.

There is also often a nice flush in fall, when the rains return. It likes the moist shoulder seasons and does not like the warm or hot months, when it disappears to make way for more drought-tolerant species. Chickweed will come back in a patch year after year, so keep track of your harvest spot.

I harvest chickweed mostly from farms and gardens where it is not wanted, making it the most sustainable type of harvest. You can even collect seeds and introduce them into a soft, moist corner of your garden. Chickweed will thrive with the addition of fresh compost and manure.

Flowers have
five V-shaped
petals.

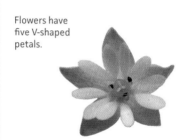

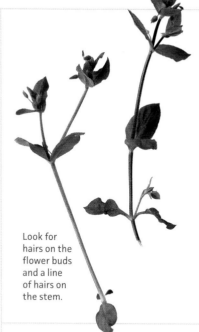

Opposite
leaves on long,
tender stems

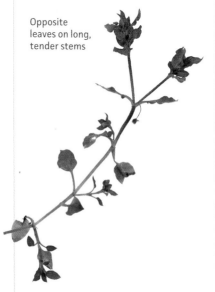

Look for
hairs on the
flower buds
and a line
of hairs on
the stem.

Chickweed has a rubber-like inner
tendon that sets it apart from
many look-alikes. Pull the stem
gently apart to reveal it.

↓

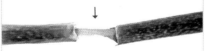

Look-Alike 🛈

Speedwell (*Veronica* spp.) has
serrations in the leaves and
purple flowers.

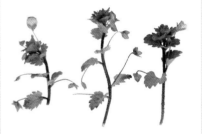

Look-Alike 🛈

Mouse-eared chickweed (*Cerastium
glomeratum*) is also edible, though not
quite as tasty as chickweed. It is covered
in short hairs.

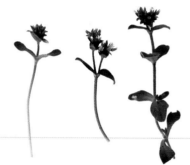

Medicinal Uses of Chickweed

You can eat chickweed, drink the tea, or use it topically. Chickweed lies on the border between medicine and food, much like hawthorn berries. Its high amount of nutrients make it particularly beneficial: it has very large amounts of vitamin C, calcium, and iron, as well as many other trace minerals and vitamins. I especially like to snack on it when I am harvesting as this is when a plant's nutrients are the highest.

Chickweed helps reduce lymphatic congestion. Like other lymphatic-mobilizing herbs, it contains a type of saponin, a compound that facilitates the flow of fluids in the body. Saponins are what makes soap slippery! This lymphatic action makes chickweed helpful for skin diseases like dermatitis, acne, and eczema. Chickweed is not a heroic remedy (meaning it is not fast acting) and requires consistent use over a period of time to make lasting change.

CHICKWEED PESTO
Makes about 1 cup

This recipe can be adapted to use many wild greens and herbs. I like to add parsley and mint from my garden, or rosemary and oregano to give it a kick. Use this as a jumping-off point and get creative! You can also add Parmesan and basil for a more classic pesto taste.

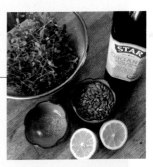

½ cup toasted sunflower seeds
4 cups tightly packed fresh chickweed
¼ cup freshly squeezed lemon juice
  (approximately 1 large lemon)
1 clove garlic
¼ teaspoon sea salt
⅓ cup organic extra-virgin olive oil

Put the seeds in the bowl of a food processor and roughly grind them into a meal.
    Add the chickweed, lemon juice, garlic, and salt and process into a paste, about 1 minute.
    Add the oil all at once, pulsing to combine.
    Serve on pasta, or just on toast!
    Store any unused pesto in a sealed container in the fridge for up to 5 days.

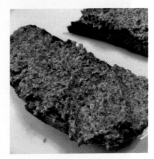

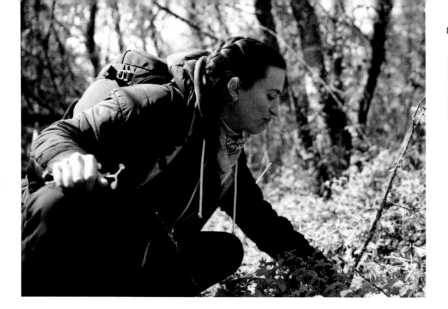

Because of its softening and decongesting action, chickweed is also used to help dissolve various types of cysts and growths. For this purpose, I would use poke (*Phytolacca* spp.) root salve topically along with the chickweed.

I like to munch on chickweed while hiking or on a stroll at a local park. (Photo by Wren Morrow)

Making Medicine with Chickweed

Chickweed is one of my favorite edible greens. It is best eaten raw, as it gets kind of slimy when cooked, much like lettuce. You can make pesto and salad with it, or use it on anything that you might put lettuce or arugula on. It has a nice mild flavor and a lovely texture.

People also use it as a poultice and as an infused oil. Keep in mind that the infused oil lasts for one year or less, as chickweed loses its medicinal properties very quickly. To make the infused oil, use fresh chickweed, leave it out to wilt for twenty-four hours, and then use the hot-water-bath method for twelve hours (see Cottonwood Bud Infused Oil).

You can also make a delightful hot infusion with fresh chickweed. I find it makes me feel generally lighter and less congested. You can also purchase dried chickweed for making tea, though it quickly loses its potency when dried and should only be kept for a year.

Cleavers

Galium aparine
Rubiaceae (bedstraw family)

Cleavers (*Galium aparine*) is an incredibly widespread plant, growing in almost every state in the US. It is considered native to the Pacific Northwest. Though we have about ten species in the genus *Galium* in Washington, cleavers is the most common and the one with the longest history of use. Be aware that there are other plants with the same whorled leaf pattern, but they typically do not stick to your clothing as aggressively as cleavers.

Some people have referred to this plant as "sticky willy," or "stickweed," because it has small barbs all over the plant that allow it to stick to clothing and hair. The seeds also have these little barbs, which they use to catch rides on animals (and human foragers), ensuring that the plant is dispersed over a wider area. How intelligent! This is a fun plant for kids to use to make costumes and crowns with the long, thin vines.

Cleavers prefers moist habitats with soft, disturbed soil. You will often find it growing alongside chickweed, nettle, horsetail, and other weedy plants that thrive in moist meadows and disturbed areas.

LEFT In some places, cleavers can cover the ground entirely, forming a thick mat. **RIGHT** Every year, I end up making a cleavers crown and wearing it for a whole day of class. There is something about this plant that brings out playfulness.

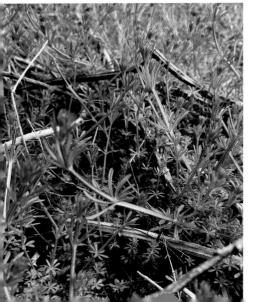
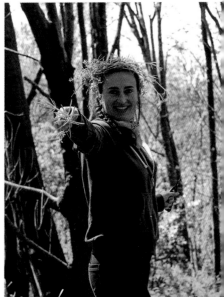

Four-petaled
white flower

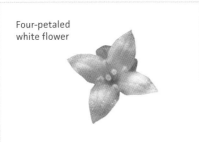

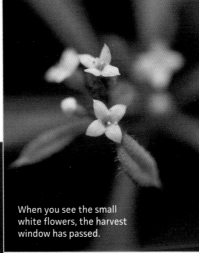

When you see the small
white flowers, the harvest
window has passed.

A pair of seeds

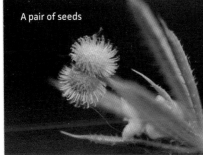

Whorled leaf
pattern

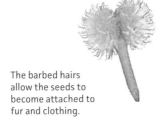

The barbed hairs
allow the seeds to
become attached to
fur and clothing.

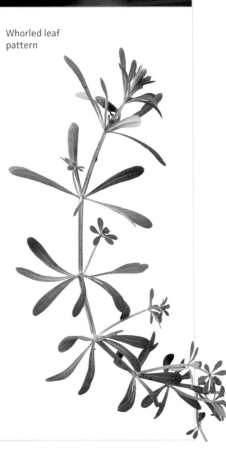

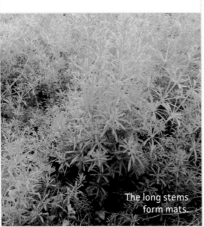

The long stems
form mats.

Harvesting Cleavers

It is best to harvest cleavers in the spring, before it flowers. This means March in most places, around the same time you harvest spring nettle and chickweed. Cut bunches of the tops, avoiding the less attractive lower parts of the plant that have brown leaves. Find cleavers growing in abundant patches in weedy, disturbed areas. I typically harvest in local parks. You may even have some growing already in your garden.

Cleavers typically flowers in May, and seeds begin maturing in June. There is sometimes a fall harvest as well, in late September and October, when the return of the rain and colder temperatures mimic spring.

Cleavers seeds do contain caffeine and can be harvested and roasted to make a caffeinated tea. However, harvesting enough seeds to drink cleavers-seed tea every morning instead of coffee would be incredibly difficult. I suppose you could send your kids to play in a field of it, then pick the seeds off their clothing!

Medicinal Uses of Cleavers

Cleavers seeds hitching a ride on a jacket while a forager harvests wild lettuce

This plant has an affinity for the pelvic area, and it is a diuretic and helps mobilize the lymphatic system. It is soothing and cooling. I use this herb to treat signs of stagnation or inflammation in the pelvic organs, which could include dark or cloudy urine, prostate inflammation, or frequent urination.

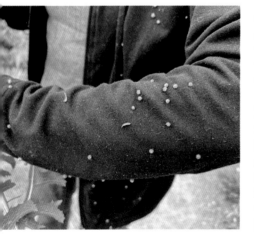

For bladder irritations, it can be combined in a tea with corn silk and marshmallow root. For prostate inflammation, try combining it with nettle root and echinacea in a tincture.

It can also be used for other problems with lymphatic stagnation. It is used in various skin disorders, including eczema, psoriasis, acne, and benign growths. For skin issues, try combining it in a tea or tincture formula with herbs such as red clover, calendula, dandelion root, yellow dock root, and burdock root.

CLEAVERS JUICE *Makes about 8 ounces*

This method of making green juice can be used with many different plants, such as chickweed, plantain, wheat grass, and parsley. Use a nut-milk bag—a fine nylon mesh bag that is used to filter the pulp out of nut milk—to strain the mixture after blending. They are sold at kitchen stores, natural food stores, and on the internet (see Resources). If you don't have a nut-milk bag, you can use a couple of layers of cheesecloth draped over a fine-mesh strainer. Chop the cleavers before blending to prevent them from getting wrapped around the blade and ruining the motor. To make the juice shelf stable, you can add ⅓ cup 190-proof alcohol to this recipe (the final product must have at least 20 percent alcohol).

Dosage: Drink in 2-ounce portions once a day.

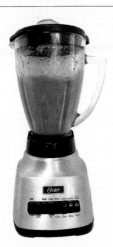

2 to 3 handfuls of fresh cleavers, roughly
   chopped
1 cup water

Add the chopped cleavers and water to a blender. Run the blender for about 30 seconds, until the mixture is a thoroughly green smoothie-like consistency.

Hold a nut-milk bag over a bowl and pour the green pulp into the bag. Once it's all in there, squeeze the bag with both hands, releasing the filtered juice through the nut-milk bag.

Transfer to a sealed glass jar and store in the fridge for no more than 3 days. To freeze the juice for future use, pour it into an ice cube tray, freeze it until solid, and then put the cubes into a labeled plastic freezer bag. The cubes will keep for 1 year in the freezer.

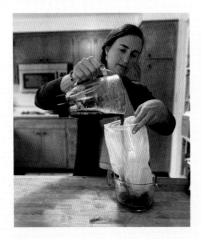

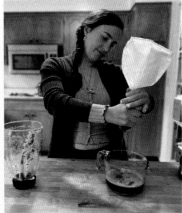

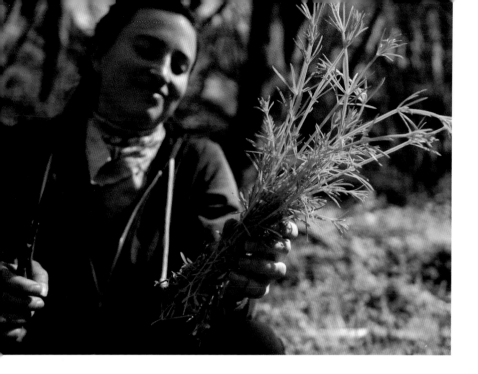

Harvesting cleavers in a bigleaf maple forest in early April (Photo by Wren Morrow)

Making Medicine with Cleavers

The most traditional preparation of cleavers is a succus, which is basically a juice preserved with alcohol. You can also just make a juice by chopping up the herb, putting it into a blender with some water, and then straining through a nut-milk bag. I use a nut-milk bag specifically because it is fine enough to catch the small barbs, which can irritate your throat if not filtered out (see Cleavers Juice recipe).

You can also dry the leaves and stems for tea. These don't keep very long—their freshness is indicated by how green they are. Store for no more than a year, as its potency diminishes quickly. It is generally believed that this plant is better used fresh, but the tea of the dried herb is effective as well. It's also easier to add to tea formulas in the dried form.

Cramp Bark

Viburnum opulus, V. edule
Adoxaceae (muskroot family)

Species of *Viburnum* have long been used for medicine in Europe and by Native groups in North America. Cramp bark (*Viburnum opulus*) is the one I harvest locally for medicine.

Two varieties of cramp bark are common in this area: the native American highbush cranberry (*V. opulus* var. *americanum*), and the non-native cramp bark, also known as European highbush cranberry (*V. opulus* var. *opulus*). These two varieties are incredibly hard to tell apart, but they have the same medicinal actions, so it isn't important to differentiate between them.

To make sure you have *Viburnum opulus* and not its close relative *Viburnum edule*, look for the stipules and glands on the leaf stems.

Harvesting Cramp Bark

To find cramp bark, look in or near a wetland area on the west side of the Cascades. You could also consider growing it in your yard!

Cramp bark, like other barks, is best harvested from thick branches during the spring or fall. When selecting which branches to harvest, I typically harvest from the most crowded

LEFT Cramp bark berries on their way to ripeness. They will turn translucent and juicy when ripe.
RIGHT Note the glands at the base of the leaf and the stipules at the base of the leaf stem.

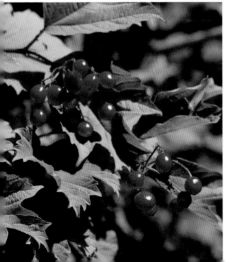
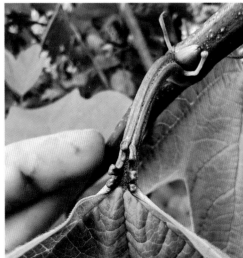

parts of the plant, with the goal of thinning it out and creating more air flow. Harvest no more than one in ten canes, which means that if there are not ten canes in the bush, don't harvest from it. Peel the bark off with a pocketknife as soon as you get home, then lay the bark out to dry. Spring bark will come off much more easily because it has more water in it.

Cramp bark is definitely one of the less common plants highlighted in this book, so be aware of your impact on the places you harvest. If you are able, consider growing it in your yard. It is very easy to propagate from a cutting harvested in the wild and grows without much interference. To aid its success, plant it in a wetter part of your yard.

Medicinal Uses of Cramp Bark

As the name suggests, cramp bark is indeed used for cramps. It is a wonderful antispasmodic, which means that it helps calm muscular spasms. It has an affinity for the pelvic area, a fact that I didn't understand until I took a large dose before bed. I felt my entire pelvic area become profoundly relaxed, almost like it was sinking into the bed itself. Wild! It will work for other areas of the body, but it will work best for pain in that area. Holding to this pelvic theme, cramp bark is used for menstrual cramps and uterine cramping in general, for pain from urinary tract infections, and also for the pain from kidney stones.

LEFT Cramp bark is a leggy shrub that grows near wetlands and lakes. RIGHT Peeling cramp bark in the field after harvesting on a sunny October day

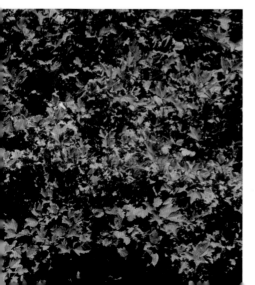
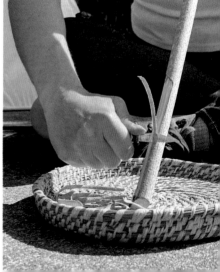

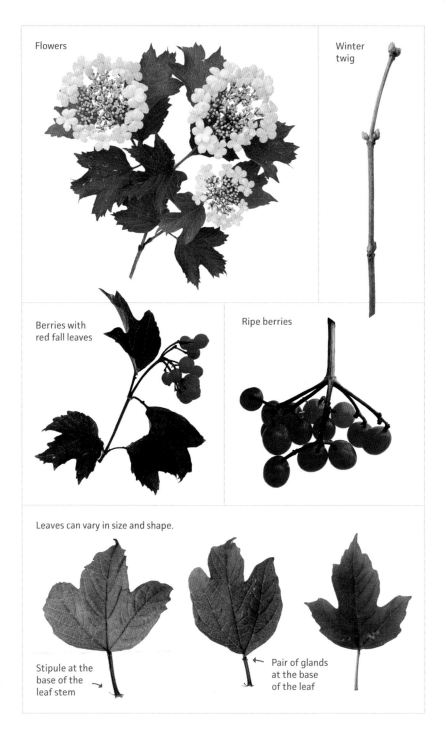

Flowers

Winter twig

Berries with red fall leaves

Ripe berries

Leaves can vary in size and shape.

Stipule at the base of the leaf stem

Pair of glands at the base of the leaf

For menstrual cramps, I combine it with motherwort. For all types of muscular spasms and pain, I combine it with willow bark.

The antispasmodic properties of cramp bark are also used to calm bronchial spasms of asthma. For this, it is typically combined with other antispasmodics, such as lobelia (*Lobelia inflata*), and expectorants like elecampane (*Inula helenium*).

You can also use cramp bark topically to soothe spasming muscles (see Antispasmodic Liniment).

Historically, cramp bark has also been used as a uterine tonic, both to keep the uterus from prolapsing and to maintain a healthy pregnancy. Consult a specialist before you start taking herbs during pregnancy.

Making Medicine with Cramp Bark

I almost always prepare and use cramp bark as a tincture. Cramp bark is usually used for acute scenarios, so its dosage tends to be small and frequent. Try 10 to 30 drops every 15 minutes.

I add vegetable glycerin to my tincture (to make 10 percent of the total volume) to help stabilize some of the tannins and prevent the goop that likes to form at the bottom of the jar. This

---

MENSTRUAL CRAMP FORMULA　　　　　　　　　　　*Makes 3 ounces*

This is my favorite cramp formula. It is best taken in frequent doses at the first sign of cramping. Motherwort is a mild sedative and is used in Chinese medicine to move blood and relieve uterine cramping. Though it doesn't grow wild where we live, it grows well in our bioregion. This formula would make a great addition to a personal herbal first aid kit.

Dosage: Take 30 to 60 drops every hour while cramping. Start with the smaller dose and work up. Stop using the tincture if you feel nauseous.

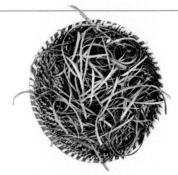

1 fluid ounce cramp bark tincture (see Tincture Ratio Chart)
1 fluid ounce motherwort tincture
1 fluid ounce willow bark tincture (see Tincture of Dried Willow Bark)

Mix all the tinctures together in a 4-ounce amber dropper bottle.
　　Store for no more than 1 year.

is a practice that some herbalists reserve for red root and horse chestnut; both contain large amounts of saponins and tannins together, which react and glom together to settle in the bottom of the jar. The tinctures of many other plants can benefit from this trick as well.

Some people make a decoction of the bark, though it has a very acrid taste that is difficult to get down.

I hear the berries make a nice jam or sauce, but I've never tried, because they do not taste great raw. Try it and let me know how it goes!

Cautions

Very large doses of cramp bark may cause nausea and vomiting.

ANTISPASMODIC LINIMENT   *Makes 3 ounces*

This is a topical formula that naturopathic doctor Nancy Welliver taught to me several years ago when I was complaining of tightness in my neck. It works like a charm. Make sure your tinctures are potent, apply often, and top with a hot cloth to make the preparation even more effective. This is for topical use only as lobelia is toxic internally. Lobelia tincture can be hard to find as not all stores sell it. You can order it online from Herb Pharm (see Resources).

Dosage: Apply to the affected area several times a day, rubbing vigorously with your hands to help it absorb into the skin. Apply a hot towel over it for even greater effects.

1 fluid ounce cramp bark tincture (see
    Tincture Ratio Chart)
1 fluid ounce St. John's wort tincture (see
    Tincture Ratio Chart)
1 fluid ounce lobelia tincture

Mix tinctures together in a glass bottle with a spray top or a roller applicator.
    The liniment will keep for up to 5 years.

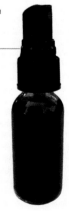

Small glass spray bottles are a great way to apply tinctures topically. Use them to spray on wrists, knees, toes, fingers, and even your neck.

Dandelion

Taraxacum officinale
Asteraceae (sunflower family)

Dandelion is a very successful weed all over the world, and it is used heavily as a food and medicine by all cultures who have it. It has a very effective seed-dispersal mechanism that helps it spread efficiently, and it is highly adaptable—able to evolve quickly depending on its growing conditions. Have you ever noticed that dandelions that grow in mown grass are flatter to the ground and smaller? That is one of the many different adaptations that dandelion has mastered.

The name comes from the French *dent de leon*, which means "lion's tooth." This comes from the lobed and serrated leaf edges that look a lot like a predator's teeth.

Harvesting Dandelion

Dandelion thriving on the edge of a gravel parking lot

Dandelion has two prominent look-alikes in our area: hairy cat's ear (*Hypochaeris radicata*) and smooth hawksbeard

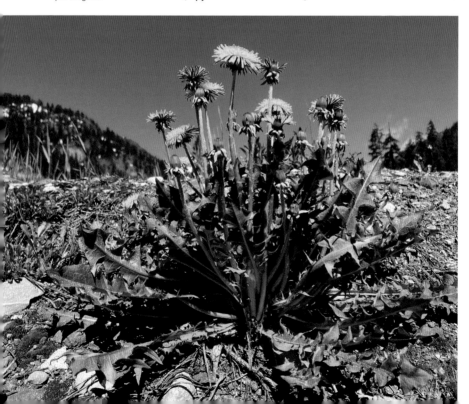

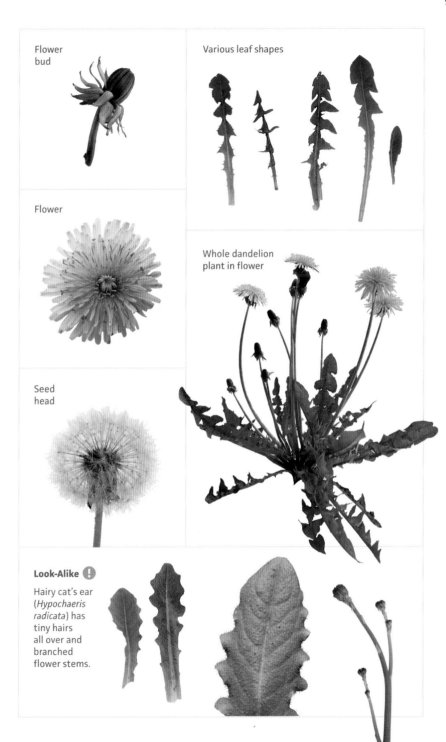

Flower bud

Various leaf shapes

Flower

Seed head

Whole dandelion plant in flower

Look-Alike

Hairy cat's ear (*Hypochaeris radicata*) has tiny hairs all over and branched flower stems.

(*Crepis capillaris*). Neither of these is toxic, and in fact both have similar edible and medicinal uses, but you want to make sure you have dandelion if that's what you're after. Other look-alikes include salsify and sow thistle, but those are much less likely to trick you.

Most commonly, people forage dandelion leaves to eat, but they also do so for medicine. The leaves are least bitter in late winter and early spring, before the plant flowers. As the plant flowers and the leaves age, they get more and more bitter, so when harvesting later in the year, select the younger, brighter leaves.

Dig the roots, which are used for food and medicine, in spring or fall, though really they can be dug anytime they are needed. I use a hori-hori knife for smaller plants or a digging fork for larger plants. You will most likely not be able to get the entire taproot of this deeply rooted plant, which means that dandelions will likely sprout from the leftover root. How sustainable! I try to select plants growing in softer mediums that will give up the roots more easily. Soft gravel, deep garden mulch, and bark chips are some of my favorite places to harvest dandelion roots.

Dandelion roots need to be thoroughly washed. I try to wash them in some way in the field, perhaps by washing them in a nearby stream, or just by knocking the dirt off as much as possible. At home, I spray them with the hose—a strong jet of water,

LEFT A dandelion seed head, a very effective seed-dispersal mechanism RIGHT Scrubbing the dirt off a dandelion root in a clean mountain stream

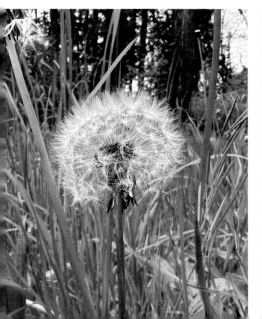
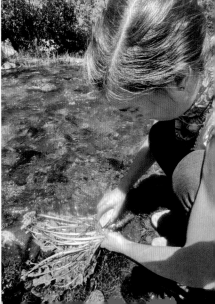

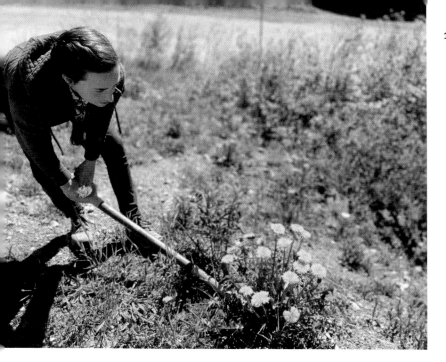

Harvesting dandelion root with a four-pronged digging fork

kind of like pressure washing. In my kitchen, I gather them all in a large metal bowl with their greens cut off and give them one last scrub. Sometimes it's necessary to cut into them to remove black or rotting parts of the root or to expose places between roots where there is still dirt.

The flower buds can be harvested to make fritters or capers. Dandelions form buds early in the year, and you will often need to hunt for them as they grow close to the crown of the plant. People also harvest dandelion flowers for making wine, beer, and soda. For this purpose, you can pick the flowers periodically and throw them in a bag in the freezer until you accumulate enough; many recipes call for a quart or more.

Medicinal Uses of Dandelion

Dandelion is bitter, cool, and draining, and it works with both the liver and kidneys. It is hard to point to a specific condition that it is good for; it simply cleans up your liver and helps you excrete stuff through urine. It can help mild constipation by stimulating liver function, it can help with skin conditions like acne and eczema by eliminating toxins in the kidneys and liver and clearing heat, and it can help with hormonal imbalance by clearing out the liver.

Dandelion root and St. John's wort bud and flower are both superstars for tempering the irritability that comes with hormonal spikes, which typically happen during ovulation and right before menstruation. This combination can also be helpful for perimenopausal and menopausal symptoms, which also involve hormone fluctuation.

I often use dandelion root when I travel, as the tea is commonly available and the plant grows in most places. When we travel, we may eat fewer vegetables and more sugary and fatty foods than we would at home. This can trigger urinary tract infections and constipation, so dandelion is a nice ally to have on hand.

For eczema and other skin conditions, dandelion root is classically combined in a formula with other detoxifying and

ROASTED DANDELION ROOTS   *Makes 1 to 2 cups of roasted roots*

Roasted dandelion root tea is a classic coffee substitute. It's not a new idea; the Japanese drank it during World War II when they could not get coffee due to trade embargoes. Now you can get it at the store. Here is one method to make it yourself from fresh dandelion roots. I drink it with milk and honey.

Dosage: Use 1 to 3 teaspoons of the roasted roots per cup of water. Simmer for about 10 minutes and strain. Drink 1 cup a day.

6 cups fresh dandelion roots,
   washed thoroughly

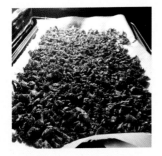

Preheat the oven to 300°F and line a baking sheet with parchment paper.

Fill the drum of a food processor with the chopped dandelion roots. Pulse until they are roughly chopped. You can also just chop them small with a knife. The pieces should be about ⅛-inch long.

Spread the dandelion roots in an even layer onto the baking sheet with as much spacing as possible and pop them into the oven.

Roast for 60 to 90 minutes, checking every 20 minutes or so to make sure they are not burning. Turn the roots a few times to promote even drying and roasting.

They will start to turn brown, and you will smell a toasty smell. You can decide how toasty you want them to be.

Remove from the oven and let cool completely. Store in a clean glass jar for up to 2 years.

cooling roots, like yellow dock, burdock, and Oregon grape. A tincture or a capsule is the preferred preparation as the flavor of these plants together is very strong. This formula can be drying, so if the formula gives you problems, switch to an eczema formula more suited to dryness. Violet leaf is a classic for that.

Dandelion leaf is used as a diuretic for folks who have edema (fluid accumulation in the feet and ankles that causes swelling). One of the benefits of dandelion leaf is that it is naturally high in potassium, a mineral that is depleted by pharmaceutical diuretics. Tea is the best way to harness the diuretic actions of this plant. You can make a tea of either the whole plant (leaf and root) or just the leaf. Keep in mind that edema can be a sign of serious illness, so please get yourself checked out by a doctor.

Dandelion, Jerusalem artichoke, and burdock all have high inulin content in their roots. Inulin is a complex starch that feeds gut bacteria in your large intestine and is considered a prebiotic. Prebiotics can help cultivate good intestinal flora over time, but consuming large amounts can cause gas and bloating. As with so many things in herbalism, it is all about the dose!

Making Medicine with Dandelion

A tincture can be made from fresh or dried dandelion root (see Tincture Ratio Chart). Having experimented with tinctures of both fresh and dried root, I prefer the dried root as it seems to be more potent. I grind up the dried dandelion root in my herb grinder to increase surface area.

A tea made from dandelion roots, either roasted or raw, is lovely (see Roasted Dandelion Roots). You can either infuse or decoct it, though decocting will get you a much stronger tea. Use between 1 teaspoon and 1 tablespoon of dried herb per cup.

Cautions

Dandelion root can be quite drying and is therefore not the best herb for someone who has a dry constitution.

Douglas-Fir

Pseudotsuga menziesii
Pinaceae (pine family)

Douglas-fir is one of the most common trees in the Pacific Northwest. It garners attention from herbalists because of its aromatic green tips that emerge in spring and its highly anti-microbial resin. Given the abundance of Douglas-fir in our region, we can harvest the tips and resin to use in medicine quite liberally.

Despite its name, Douglas-fir is not considered to be a true fir. It is in a different genus and has different bark, cones, and needles than true firs (*Abies* spp.).

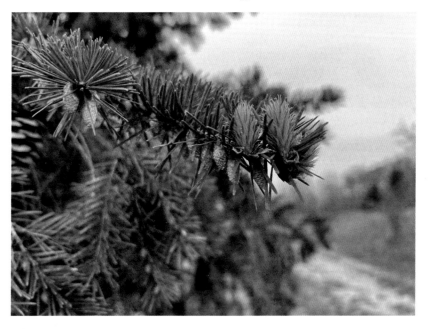

Pollen-bearing structures (orange) and flowers that will become cones (light green)

Harvesting Douglas-Fir

I love to harvest Douglas-fir tips. Harvest the bright-green new growth from the tips of the branches in spring. The green tips begin to emerge in April, typically, and can be harvested into June. The smaller tips contain fewer astringent and bitter compounds, but I harvest the tips when they are about 2 inches long because I can harvest less for more yield.

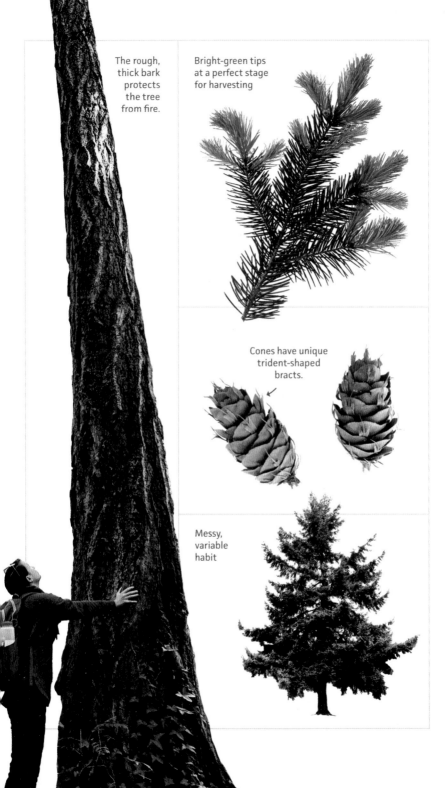

The rough, thick bark protects the tree from fire.

Bright-green tips at a perfect stage for harvesting

Cones have unique trident-shaped bracts.

Messy, variable habit

Harvesting Douglas-fir resin, on the other hand, is a sticky endeavor, so prepare yourself. Bring a piece of parchment paper to harvest into—it has a coating that prevents resin from sticking to it. The resin is the white or amber stuff that drips down the trunk and hardens as it ages. Resin seeps out of tree wounds much like a human wound would scab over. It protects the tree's wound from microbes and insects. Never remove resin directly from where it seals a wound in the bark, as that will open it up to diseases; harvest only from the excess that drips down the trunk.

If the resin is dry, you can pick it off with your fingers. If it is still sticky and wet, use a butter knife or a stick to scrape it off and avoid getting it on your fingers. No matter how careful you are, you will still likely get some sticky resin on your fingers during a harvest. You can remove this insipidly sticky stuff from your fingers with alcohol or oil, though I just cover it with silt and then rub it off, as I am often in the middle of a long hike when I find a good spot to harvest. (I've been teased for "washing my hands with dirt," but it is quite effective!) Avoid getting the resin on your clothing, as it can be incredibly difficult to remove. The resin is very shelf stable and can be stored for hundreds of years. I keep a jar into which I make small deposits of resin, which add up to a large amount over time.

Douglas-fir is so abundant in our area that there are few concerns with overharvesting. However, try to harvest where the trees are actually abundant, which isn't true of every area

LEFT Harvesting Douglas-fir tips at a local park in May (Photo by Wren Morrow) **RIGHT** Harvesting Douglas-fir resin with a butter knife and parchment paper

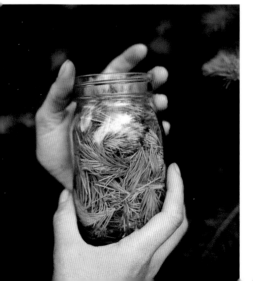
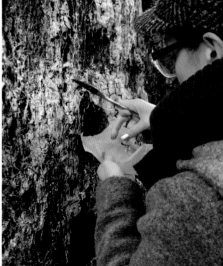

in the Pacific Northwest, such as places east of the Cascades, where ponderosa pines dominate and Douglas-firs are a rare find. And avoid harvesting the tips from very small trees, as you are robbing an entire year of growth. Instead, harvest from larger trees and distribute your picking throughout the tree and to surrounding trees.

Medicinal Uses of Douglas-Fir

Douglas-fir tips contain vitamin C, aromatic oils, antioxidants, and tannins. They are expectorant (make you cough), antimicrobial (kill microbes), antioxidant, and immune stimulating.

Douglas-fir tips are most notable for their antimicrobial and expectorant effects on the respiratory system. They are great in combination with other herbs as a tonic to help ward off colds and flus. A hot tea of Douglas-fir tips with honey is also a great cough remedy to loosen phlegm and discourage bacterial infection. I add yarrow flowers and red root flowers to this concoction, and often make this for myself while camping on the eastern slope of the Cascades in June and July, when all three of these plants are harvestable and camping season is at its best.

I also like to use Douglas-fir tips as a tincture for throat sprays. For this, you can mix Douglas-fir tincture with poplar bud and usnea tinctures for a nice antimicrobial blend. For a soothing throat spray, you could add mullein and plantain tinctures instead. I always add honey to my throat sprays as it is both soothing and antimicrobial, and it helps the herbs stick to your throat.

The resin of all trees in the pine family is highly antimicrobial. A salve made from Douglas-fir resin is great for use on cuts, acne, ingrown hairs, and even cat scratches to discourage infection. It would also be a good addition to a first aid kit. Pine resin oil can also be used for arthritic joints, probably because it is actually a bit irritating and thus increases circulation and can relieve pain caused by stagnant blood flow. A little dash of pine resin oil can help preserve other salves and creams too. I avoid using any pine resin internally, because it is so irritating to tissues (see Cautions).

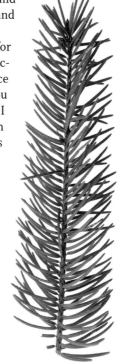

All pine resins are quite flammable, so you can mix it with dry grass to make a very nice fire starter. It has also been used as a sealant and glue for things like sealing water containers and affixing arrowheads to shafts.

DOUGLAS-FIR INFUSED VINEGAR *Makes about 12 ounces*

Infused vinegars made with aromatic herbs or berries are a delicious culinary treat. They can be added to salad dressings, marinades, or any recipe in which you'd use vinegar. Douglas-fir vinegar is lemony and sweet with a hint of pine. The vinegar extracts and preserves the vitamin C in fir tips quite well. Try using champagne vinegar, white wine vinegar, or rice vinegar in place of the apple cider vinegar. Any tree in the pine family can be used in this recipe. I harvest the tips directly into the jar so I know exactly how much I need.

About 2 cups Douglas-fir tips, enough
    to fill a 16-ounce jar
1½ to 2 cups apple cider vinegar

Chop the tips on a cutting board using clippers or a knife. Chopping will make for a stronger extraction by opening up more surface area. Put the fir tips in a clean 16-ounce jar.

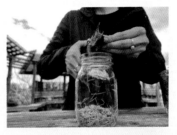

Pour the vinegar over the top until it covers the fir tips. Remember that using less liquid and more plant material creates a stronger product.

Use a plastic lid to seal the jar, shake well, and store in a cool, dark place. Let sit for about 2 weeks. Shake it a few times during this period.

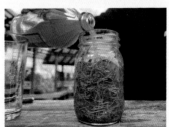

When it's finished infusing, strain through cheesecloth or a nut-milk bag, squeezing to get the flavor out of the tips. If you taste it and decide you would like it to be stronger, feel free to add another batch of fresh tips to the strained vinegar and let sit for another 2 weeks.

Store it in a glass bottle with a plastic lid in the cabinet to use in cooking. I use an old vinegar bottle for mine.

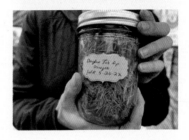

Making Medicine with Douglas-Fir

Fresh Douglas-fir tips can be steeped in cold water in the fridge overnight to make a refreshing cold-infused tea. You can also steep the tips in hot water for ten to fifteen minutes in a teapot. Knowing how much to use depends on how strong you like your tea. Start with a handful in a quart-size vessel and try it. When you are out hiking, put some in your water bottle to add a refreshing taste to your water.

Douglas-fir tips have a bright, sweet, lemony flavor that I love to capture in various preparations, which I use more for enjoyment than for medicine, to be honest. Douglas-fir syrup is a favorite, and for that I recommend double-macerating it (see the Double Maceration section in the Making Medicine chapter).

Douglas-fir oxymel is nice because it is shelf stable. It is made by making a 1:1 mix of vinegar and honey and macerating chopped Douglas-fir tips in it for two to four weeks. Oxymels, very close to shrubs, another type of vinegar-based syrup, are a cough remedy first mentioned in ancient Greek medical texts. See the Douglas-Fir Infused Vinegar recipe, which can easily be modified to make an oxymel by replacing half the vinegar with honey. Use it straight to treat a cough or sore throat. Oxymels also happen to be delicious in soda water as a mocktail.

Cautions

Resin from pine-family trees, including Douglas-fir, should not be taken internally in doses exceeding 30 drops of standardized tincture in one day, as it can result in kidney damage or joint pain. Use caution even when taking small amounts, such as 10 drops of the tincture. Historical accounts refer to pine resin being used internally, but that does not necessarily mean it is safe. Do not take pine bark internally for long periods or in large doses.

Elder

Sambucus racemosa, S. cerulea
Adoxaceae (moschatel family)

We have two native species of elder that are used for medicine in this region: red elder (*Sambucus racemosa*) and blue elder (*Sambucus cerulea*). Most commercial elderberry products are made from black elder (*Sambucus nigra*), which grows wild in Europe. Its berries are much darker than either of our species. You can easily grow black elder in your yard, but it does not grow in the wild here.

Red elder grows in forests and wet fields on the west side of the Cascades and especially thrives on the Washington and Oregon coasts. I have a keen memory of driving to the ocean late at night and seeing the glowing white blooms of vast red elder bushes reaching over the road and up into the sky.

Blue elder thrives especially on the eastern slope of the Cascades, but also in other eastern forests and fields throughout the region. It tends to need some precipitation, so you won't find it in the middle of a sagebrush steppe. You may occasionally find it west of the Cascades.

LEFT A blue elder bush on the side of the highway **RIGHT** Blue elder harvest in September in eastern Washington

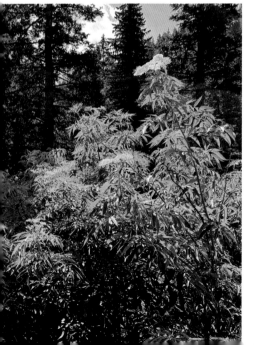
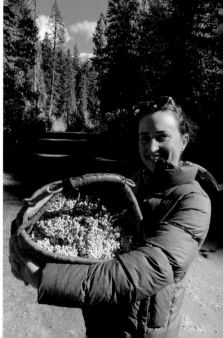

Red elder
Sambucus racemosa

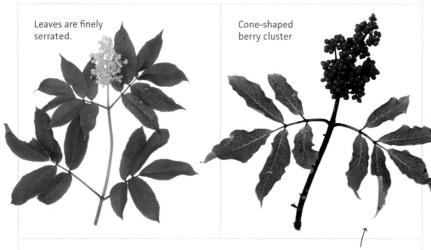

Leaves are finely serrated.

Cone-shaped berry cluster

Pinnately compound leaf arrangement

Blue elder
Sambucus cerulea

Blue elder leaves are sometimes pinnately compound and sometimes bipinnately compound.

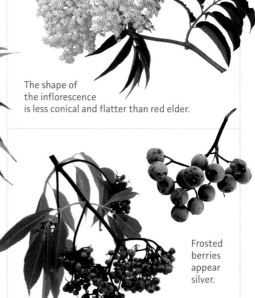

The shape of the inflorescence is less conical and flatter than red elder.

Bipinnately compound leaf

Frosted berries appear silver.

Harvesting Elder

The flowers of red elder bloom early in the year, starting in March at sea level and ending in July high up in the mountains. They are easily distinguished from blue elder by the shape of the flower clusters.

Blue elder begins blooming in May and blooms through August. These flowers are preferable to red elder for making elderflower cordials and such because their flavor and smell are more like the classic European black elder. Snip the flower heads off just as they are opening and the most aromatic. If you lean in to smell the flower, some pollen might come off on your nose. Elderflowers often have a lot of small beetles and bugs crawling around them, so leave your collection bag open for a while to allow the bugs to escape.

The berries of red elder are harvested less often because of their reputation as being toxic. Some folks go ahead and make syrup and jellies from them anyway. They do have a greater amount of the same toxic compounds that blue and black elder have, so cook well and don't eat too many. Because of its early bloom, red elder also fruits much earlier, starting in early July. You can snip the whole cluster off, just as you would harvest grapes.

Blue elderberries are the elderberry of choice in our area. They are ripe in September and October—the huge, fat berries weigh down the branches of the bushes quite heavily. Choose the darker berries—with their frosted skin, it can be difficult

LEFT Harvest ripe blue elderberries by snipping off the clusters, as you would grapes.
RIGHT Harvest the flower heads of blue elder in the spring. Avoid tugging on the breakable branches of elder, which can be tempting when flowers are high up.

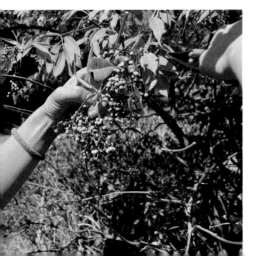

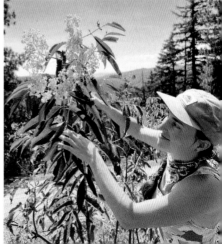

to tell when they are ripe, but if you wipe some off with your finger, you should see purple and not green underneath. Snip off whole clusters with scissors, being careful not to bend the breakable branches too much when trying to get clusters that are higher up. I harvest a lot and freeze them in clusters for projects throughout the year. Frozen elderberries are very easy to get off the stems.

Medicinal Uses of Elder

Though elderflower and elderberry have some similar effects, their uses are pretty different. Elderflower is very cooling in nature, which is why elderflower cordial is a popular summer

---

ELDERFLOWER SYRUP   *Makes 12 to 16 ounces*

Elderflower syrup and elderflower cordial are very common in Europe, where they are used in cocktails, sodas, lemonades, and sometimes desserts. This elderflower syrup is floral, sweet, and sour, and really quenches your thirst on a hot summer day. Add ¼ cup to a glass of ice and soda water for a nice refreshing beverage. The optional vodka or brandy will extend the shelf life of the syrup, or you can double the sugar to preserve it for longer.

2 cups fresh blue or red elderflowers
1 small lemon, sliced
1 cup granulated cane sugar
1 cup water
1 tablespoon vodka or brandy (optional)

Remove most of the stems from the elderflowers. Loosely pack them into a clean 16-ounce jar with the lemon slices.

Combine the sugar and water in a medium saucepan and warm on medium heat until the sugar is dissolved, about 1 to 2 minutes. Do not leave this on the stove or the sugar will burn.

Pour the hot simple syrup over the elderflowers and let sit for 4 to 6 hours with the lid resting loosely on top.

Strain the syrup using a piece of cheesecloth or a fine-mesh strainer. Add the optional vodka or brandy.

Store in a glass bottle or jar in the fridge. The syrup will last 1 to 6 months in the fridge, depending on whether you add the alcohol and how much sugar you use. It will eventually grow mold, so if it shows signs of spoiling, do not consume and discard it.

beverage all over Europe. The flower contains a large amount of quercetin and some other anti-inflammatory compounds that make it useful for hay fever and other allergic responses. It is commonly found in herbal formulas alongside nettle, goldenrod, and eyebright. It is used to help clear skin ailments like rashes or other itchy red skin conditions and can be combined with herbs like burdock for this purpose.

The flower can also calm vascular inflammation along with plants like hawthorn. The flower is also a fantastic diaphoretic (induces sweat), making it a great herb to help break a fever. For this, consider combining it with yarrow or boneset.

Elderberry is primarily used as an immune tonic and antiviral. Elderberry syrup is a popular preventative treatment during cold and flu season for both kids and adults. It can also

BLUE ELDERBERRY SYRUP   *Makes 2 to 3 cups*

Elderberry syrup is a popular immune remedy that is often taken by the spoonful daily during cold and flu season. You can also drink it with soda water or use it on pancakes. The optional brandy or vodka will increase the shelf life of your syrup, or you can double the sugar to preserve it for longer.

3 cups water
1 cup fresh blue elderberries, or
 ½ cup dried blue elderberries
½-inch piece of fresh ginger,
 thinly sliced
1 cinnamon stick
1 to 1½ cups granulated
 cane sugar
1 tablespoon brandy or vodka
 (optional)

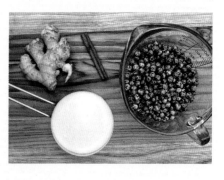

Add the water, elderberries, ginger, and cinnamon to a medium saucepan and bring to a boil over high heat. Turn the heat down to low and simmer for about 30 minutes, or until the liquid has reduced by half.

Strain through a fine-mesh strainer into a glass measuring cup to measure the liquid. Add the same volume of sugar as the liquid: if you have 1½ cups of liquid, add 1½ cups of sugar. Add the optional brandy or vodka.

Stir thoroughly and pour into a clean glass jar or bottle. Keep in the fridge.

The syrup will last 1 to 6 months in the fridge, depending on whether you add the alcohol and how much sugar you use. It will eventually grow mold, so if it shows signs of spoiling, do not consume and discard it.

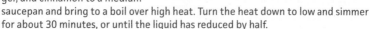

be taken at the beginning stages of a cold or flu to help fight off the virus.

The leaves and bark of elder have historically been used for medicine, though they are used less commonly now. Because those parts of the plant contain more of the toxic compound, they were used to induce vomiting (see Cautions). The practice of inducing vomiting in patients was a lot more common in the past, especially in European herbal traditions, and is not practiced often nowadays in the US.

Making Medicine with Elder

Elderflower is typically consumed as a tincture (see Tincture Ratio Chart) or as a tea of the dried flowers. Elderflower cordial or syrup is delicious. The flowers are quite hard to dry without becoming moldy, so I typically buy dried elderflowers for tea. If you are going to dry them yourself, try the blue elderflowers as they don't have the weird smell that the red elderflowers do, and they are less moist.

Because heat destroys the toxic compounds, elderberry syrup is the most common preparation of the berries (see Blue Elderberry Syrup). You can also make a tincture of the fresh or dried berries (see Tincture Ratio Chart), but be aware that it will make some sensitive folks nauseous (see Cautions). Other common preparations include elderberry oxymel, elderberry cordial, and elderberry jelly. Berries of the blue elder can take a long time to dry, so use a dehydrator if possible.

Cautions

All species of *Sambucus* can cause nausea and vomiting due to the presence of cyanogenic glycosides; some species have more than others. Different parts of the plant contain more of the compounds: The seeds contain the most, then the bark, then the leaves. The flowers and berries contain the least. These compounds are destroyed by heat.

Fennel

Foeniculum vulgare
Apiaceae (carrot family)

Fennel has an incredibly wide range where it grows wild and can grow in many different climates. It originates from the Mediterranean, which is why fennel so often appears in the cuisines of Italy, Greece, Turkey, and other countries in that region.

Common fennel has naturalized here in the Pacific Northwest. It is most commonly found growing along roadsides and in open disturbed land, such as vacant lots, pastures, and farms. It is considered a Class B noxious weed in several counties in western Washington due to its threat to native grasslands. When fennel gets established, it does tend to get aggressive and can be very difficult to remove. I have seen it pushing up sidewalks in Seattle. This makes fennel a very sustainable harvest.

The flower clusters of fennel, as with other carrot-family plants, are arranged in the shape of an upside-down umbrella, which we call an *umbel*. Fennel can be mistaken for poisonous carrot-family members like poison hemlock, but there are two key distinctions: First, the flowers of fennel are yellow, while the flowers of poison hemlock are white. Second, the leaves of fennel are not flat. Like dill, fennel has wirelike leaves. Poison

LEFT In spring, the tender green leaves of fennel grow up through the brown stalks from the previous year. **RIGHT** Fennel, being a Mediterranean plant, seems to like growing near pavement because of the extra warmth it provides.

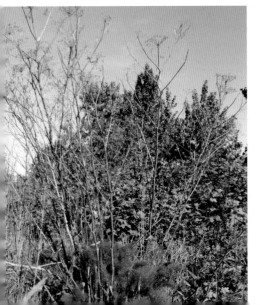
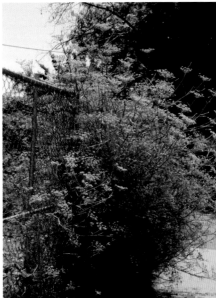

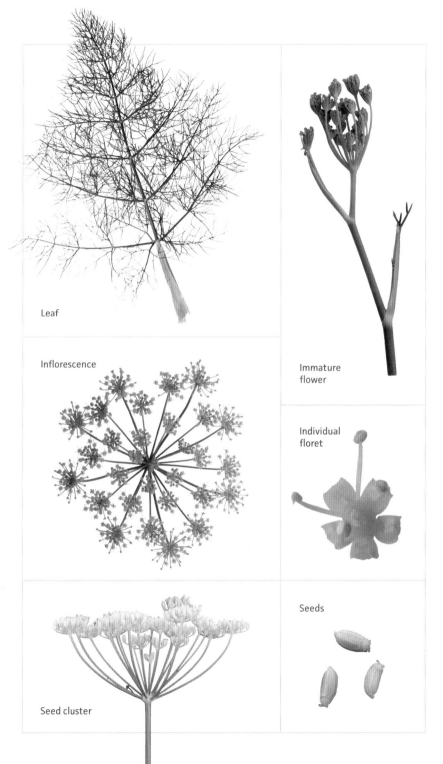

Leaf

Inflorescence

Immature flower

Individual floret

Seeds

Seed cluster

hemlock has flat leaves, more like flat-leaf parsley (see the Poison Hemlock entry in Part Three: Poisonous and Toxic Plants).

There are many varieties of fennel that have been bred by humans for different flavors, so if you want to grow it in your garden, there are many choices. The seeds of the wild type are not as sweet as those you'll find in the spice aisle at the store, but it is strongly aromatic, a little bitter, and a little spicy. I quite like it! The plant is a perennial; the aboveground parts die off in the winter and then sprout up the next year from the same root stock.

Harvesting Fennel

For medicine, we mostly use the seeds. The seeds are best harvested when they are immature, plump, and blue green. They are sweeter and more aromatic at that stage than when they dry out. Not to mention that if you wait too long to harvest in a rainy climate, they may rot rather than dry. The seeds begin maturing as early as June and may be found as late as October. Aphids and other bugs are quite fond of the seeds, so earlier harvests are more bug-free.

I harvest the entire umbel and dry them whole. Once they are fully dry, I pull the seeds off with my fingers and store them in a glass jar, discarding the stems.

The leaves can be eaten in salads, the new and tender ones being the best for harvest. These begin to emerge in March and are in full swing in May. You can find several nice Italian recipes using fennel leaves.

The bulb and stalk of cultivated fennel are eaten, but the wild one is a bit too fibrous for that. However, the stalks are hollow inside, so you could make a drinking straw if you are feeling fancy.

Medicinal Uses of Fennel

Fennel is quite useful and versatile medicinally. It is first and foremost a digestive herb, helping to ease gas and spasms in the intestines and aid peristalsis (the muscular process of moving things along in your intestines). The word for this is *carminative*. There are many familiar carminatives in the carrot family, such as coriander, dill, caraway, and cumin. Fennel can also be used for general indigestion and for poor absorption. I like to drink fennel tea or chew on a few fennel seeds as a post-meal digestive aid.

Fennel and anise seeds are a popular ingredient in aperitifs and digestifs, which are herb-infused liqueurs consumed before or after mealtimes in Europe. There is a long tradition in Europe of complex herbal recipes for these concoctions that are diligently kept secret. See the Fennel Digestif recipe to prepare your own to sip after meals.

Because of fennel's aromatic properties, it opens the lungs and aids breathing, making it useful in asthma formulas. It is also beneficial for phlegmy coughs, helping to thin and expel mucus.

Fennel seeds have long been used to encourage milk production while breastfeeding. For this, it is often combined with fenugreek seed in a daily tea.

Fennel is also beneficial for the liver and is used for jaundice and other liver issues. The seeds can also be used as a tea to reduce bladder inflammation.

When in full bloom, fennel is full of pollinators, including wasps, beetles, and bees of all kinds.

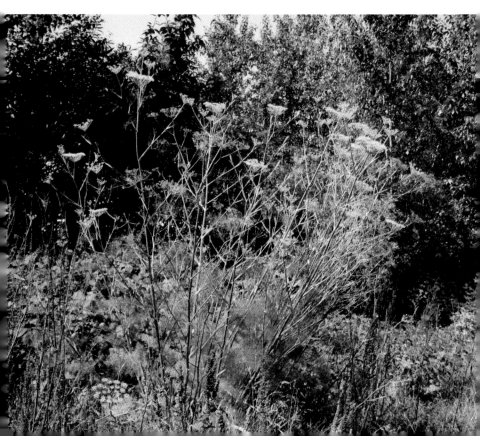

Making Medicine with Fennel

Fennel is typically consumed as a hot infusion of the seeds. Use 1 tablespoon of seeds per cup for a strong brew. You can also make a tincture of the seeds (see Tincture Ratio Chart). To make a stronger tincture, grind the dried seeds or crush the fresh seeds to increase the surface area.

Fennel also makes a delicious glycerite. A glycerite uses vegetable glycerin, a liquid solvent that is thick and sweet tasting and is often used in place of alcohol for populations that prefer to avoid alcohol.

You can use fennel in infused liqueurs, in combination with other herbs and spices (see the Fennel Digestif recipe).

Fennel seed is also a common culinary herb and can be used in spice blends, soups, homemade sausage, and more.

FENNEL DIGESTIF   *Makes 12 ounces*

This carminative after-dinner liqueur comes from a long-standing European tradition of drinking herb-infused alcohol before or after meals to improve digestion. They are served in tiny cordial glasses and sipped slowly over good conversation. Any number of other herbs and spices may be added. Be creative! The alcohol is very strong, so serve in 1-ounce portions.

---

2 tablespoons fresh or dried fennel seed
4 tablespoons granulated cane sugar
2 teaspoons fresh orange zest (from an
   organic orange)
1½ cups 80-proof alcohol (40 percent),
   such as vodka

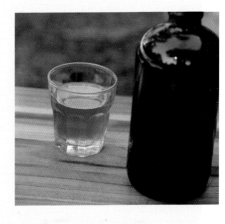

If you are using fresh fennel seeds, crush them a bit with your fingers or a mortar and pestle before adding them to a 16-ounce mason jar.

Add the sugar and orange zest and pour the vodka over the top.

Seal the jar with the lid and shake it well, until all the sugar has dissolved. Label well.

Let the jar sit in a cool, dark place for 4 weeks.

Strain using a cheesecloth over a fine-mesh metal strainer, and store in a pretty bottle for up to 5 years.

Fir

Abies grandis, A. amabilis, A. procera, A. lasiocarpa
Pinaceae (pine family)

There are four main species of fir in the Pacific Northwest: grand fir (*Abies grandis*), Pacific silver fir (*Abies amabilis*), noble fir (*Abies procera*), and subalpine fir (*Abies lasiocarpa*). Grand fir and Pacific silver fir are the most abundant, so these are the ones I harvest. Avoid harvesting from subalpine fir because it has a limited habitat and a very slow growth rate.

Firs are easy to distinguish from other members of the pine family, like Douglas-fir, because the cones of all species sit on top of the branch and point upward. However, fir cones can be difficult to spot because they grow at the very top of the tree. When I was on the ski lift as a kid, I could see the Pacific silver fir cones pointing up at me from the treetops below. The cones are often ripped apart by squirrels, who love to eat the nuts hidden between the scales, leaving only the pointy, central stem and a mess of scales strewn about. You can often find piles of these scales at the base of fir trees.

Grand fir is my favorite among the evergreen trees in our area because it smells and tastes absolutely delectable. It is much less common than Douglas-fir but well worth tracking down. I have the best luck finding it in the Cascades on both sides and around the Puget Sound. Many parks also plant grand fir, often

LEFT A grand fir tree against a backdrop of black cottonwoods **RIGHT** Fir cones grow upward, and open up to drop seed on hot days.

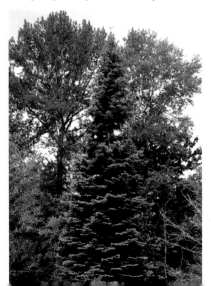
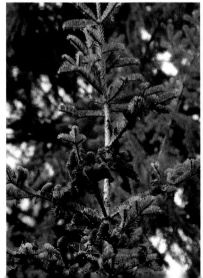

Pacific silver fir
Abies amabilis

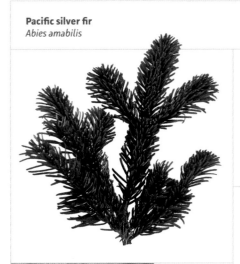

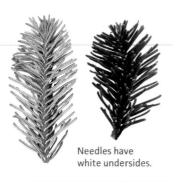

Needles have white undersides.

Fir cones always point upward and are found at the top of the tree.

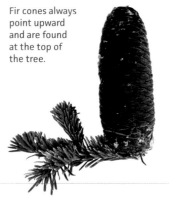

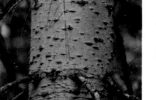

Most fir species have resin-filled pockets in the bark.

Grand fir
Abies grandis

Grand fir is very full, and branches tend to point upward. (Photo by Craig Althen)

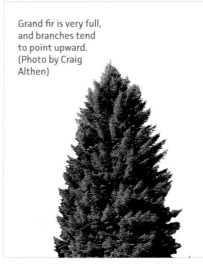

Needles lie flat.

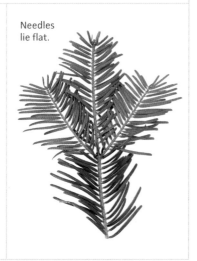

in restoration areas where they are introducing native plants. I have also seen a lot in the Columbia Gorge.

Pacific silver fir typically grows at higher elevations (at 1,000 to 4,000 feet), and thus is found in the Cascades of Washington and Oregon and in the Olympics. It is also found around the Gulf Islands in Canada and up the coast almost to Alaska. This fir has a silver tint to the underside of its needles, making it easy to spot among other evergreens.

Harvesting Fir

Grand fir tips are ready for harvest at sea level in mid-May, and more like June or July at higher elevations. Pacific silver fir tips, because of their higher-elevation location, emerge in June or July, depending on the elevation and which direction the slope is facing. South-facing slopes get more sun and thus the tips emerge earlier.

Some folks like to harvest the tips when they first emerge because they are sweeter at this stage, and that's a good call if you are making something to consume that retains the actual plant material in the final product, like an herbal salt or sugar. However, for most other preparations, I harvest fir tips when they are 2 to 3 inches in length. This allows me to harvest fewer

LEFT Pluck the tender, bright-green new growth off, avoiding trees that are too young. (Photo by Wren Morrow) **RIGHT** Harvesting grand fir needles while ski touring in the Cascades

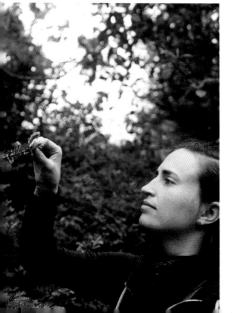
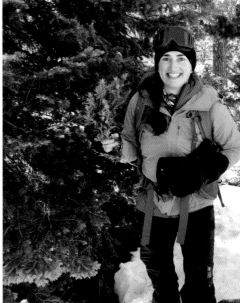

tips overall, which takes less time and has less of an impact on the tree's growth.

Fir resin—a sticky substance that is created by trees to protect wounds from pathogens and insect invasion—is very medicinal and can be harvested by picking the glass-like drops off the sides of the tree. Try to find resin that's as dry as possible; harvesting resin that's still sticky is a messy ordeal. Harvest directly into a parchment-paper bag or onto a piece of waxed paper. In a pinch, you can harvest into a plastic bag or glass jar, but keep in mind that it will stick. The resin easily ruins clothing and sticks in hair, so take care when harvesting. Please avoid harvesting from wounds or branch scars, where you might remove the protective resin coating and expose the wound to pathogens.

Fir needles can be harvested at any stage of growth, though they develop more astringent compounds as they mature. The stem especially tastes astringent, so remove the needles to use and discard the stem. They have the same medicinal uses as the tips.

Medicinal Uses of Fir

Fir trees have a long history of use in herbal medicine all around the world. You will find firs in any herbal tradition that had access to them. Nicholas Culpeper included two types of fir in his book *Complete Herbal*, published in 1653. Dioscorides, Greek physician and author of *De materia medica*, published in the first century, claimed to prefer fir resin over other types of resin because it is so clear and sweet smelling.

Fir tips are antimicrobial, expectorant, and very high in vitamin C, making them a great herb for preventing and treating winter coughs. You will see fir essential oil commonly used in aromatic chest rubs, along with camphor, eucalyptus, and menthol crystals.

Fir resin is used much like the resins from other trees in the pine family (see the Spruce entry, for example). These resins are used medicinally mainly because the resins and volatile oils kill microbes and

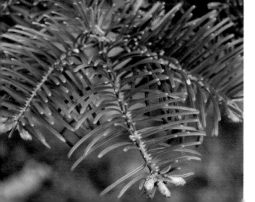

Grand fir needles

promote circulation. Fir resin can be used as a salve or oil on cuts to prevent or treat minor infections.

Tree resins also have a history of use for stomach ulcers, probably due to their antimicrobial action. Antimicrobials are often used in the treatment of ulcers because there can be a bacterial infection involved—like *Helicobacter pylori*. Fir resin has also been used to treat drippy coughs as it is expectorant in addition to its antimicrobial properties. However, these uses are no longer favored, as tree resins can cause kidney damage and joint pain—due to their pro-inflammatory nature—when taken internally in too large a dose. I prefer to use fir tips for coughs for this reason.

Fir bark is rarely used medicinally today, and I have not used it myself, but it has a history of use among the temperate, mountain, and boreal peoples who have access to fir trees. The resin (as with all pine-family resins) has also been used traditionally by many groups for sealing containers and in glues.

FIR TIP ELIXIR   *Makes 8 ounces*

Elixirs are made with half sugar or honey and half alcohol. They are sweet and can be used in beverages or taken by the teaspoon. Feel free to swap out the sugar for honey in this recipe, though you'll want to make sure the honey is fully dissolved in the solution.

1 cup fresh fir tips
½ cup granulated cane sugar
½ cup vodka or brandy

Chop the fir tips carefully and pack loosely into a clean 16-ounce jar.

Add the sugar and vodka or brandy to the jar.

Put the lid on and shake thoroughly, until all the sugar is dissolved.

Label the jar clearly and let sit for 4 weeks in a cool, dark place. Shake a few times while it sits.

Strain, return to the original jar, and store for up to 5 years.

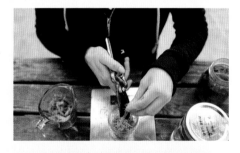
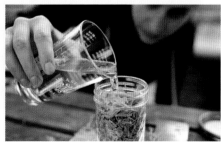

Photos by
Wren Morrow

Making Medicine with Fir

The flavor of fir reminds me of Christmas because my family always gets noble fir trees. It is deeply comforting, sweet, and nostalgic. For this reason, fir is one of my favorite evergreens to work with.

Making an infused honey, elixir, or oxymel with grand fir tips is my preferred way to prepare this herb. The oxymel makes a great mocktail. Just blend it with some club soda and ice. You can also infuse vinegars with fir tips and add those vinegars to salad dressings and other recipes (see Douglas-Fir Infused Vinegar).

A cold infusion of fresh fir tips is quite simple and absolutely delightful. Leave the tips to infuse in a jar of water in the fridge overnight and strain in the morning. It's like flavored water! Fir tips can also be dried for use in hot infusions (tea). Be sure to cover your tea so the volatile oils (the yummy-smelling part) don't evaporate. Use up any dried fir tips within one year because they don't keep their medicinal properties well.

You can use fir tips or needles to prepare a tincture (see Tincture Ratio Chart), which makes a great addition to a throat spray or cold and flu tonic.

Aromatic and sweet fir resin can be applied directly to wounds as an antimicrobial and sealant. The resin can also be melted into a carrier oil, making a great addition to salves, oils, and creams. The resin is incredibly sticky and cannot be washed off with water, so remove it from your skin with alcohol or oil.

Cautions

Resin from pine-family trees, including fir, should not be taken internally in doses exceeding 30 drops of standardized tincture in one day, as it can result in kidney damage or joint pain. Use caution even when taking small amounts, such as 10 drops of the tincture. Historical accounts refer to pine resin being used internally, but that does not necessarily mean it is safe. Do not take pine bark internally for long periods or in large doses.

Goldenrod

Solidago lepida
Asteraceae (sunflower family)

Goldenrod is surprisingly abundant in our region. Our main local species, called western Canada goldenrod (*Solidago lepida*), is native and grows in a wide range of ecosystems. We have other species too, but none of them are nearly as common. I've found it in particular abundance up on treeless mountain hillsides and meadows in the Cascades. It is a plant that seems to love growing in clear-cuts, postavalanche wastelands, and vacant lots.

One of goldenrod's look-alikes is fireweed (*Chamaenerion angustifolium*), which is vastly different once in bloom. Fireweed has fuchsia flowers that are much larger, and it does not have any teeth or serrations on its leaves. Goldenrod's closest look-alike is San Juan mugwort (*Artemisia suksdorfii*), which sometimes grows alongside it and has similar toothlike lobes on its leaves. Both are in the sunflower family, so the flower morphology is pretty similar too.

Some might confuse it with tansy (*Tanacetum vulgare*), which typically grows nearby, but once you've really looked at the two, you won't confuse them. Look up pictures online so you can see the differences.

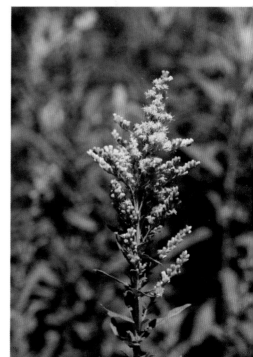

Goldenrod in full bloom

Harvesting Goldenrod

To find a goldenrod patch, I typically meander forest service roads at middle elevations on both the west and east sides of the Cascades. The goldenrod that grows on the east side of the Cascades is particularly aromatic—as are all plants that grow in drier climates. Once you find a good patch, you can return year after year to harvest, keeping tabs on its bloom time every year, which typically varies by a few days or a week depending on the weather that season.

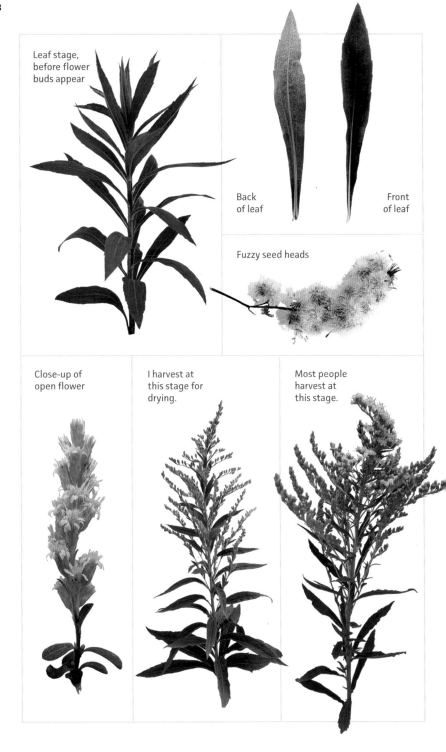

Leaf stage, before flower buds appear

Back of leaf

Front of leaf

Fuzzy seed heads

Close-up of open flower

I harvest at this stage for drying.

Most people harvest at this stage.

Goldenrod starts to flower in early July and may be blooming into August at elevation. To harvest the flowering tops, use scissors or clippers to snip off the top 5 inches, which should include the entire flower head. After drying, you can break it up further for better mixing into tea blends.

It is particularly important to harvest goldenrod flowers just as they are opening. They will look yellow before they start to open, and you can even harvest them at this bud stage. Once one or two little yellow tufts start to peek out, it's the perfect time. If you wait until they are in full flower, they will go to seed while drying and turn into fluff, much like a dandelion seed head. This is a defense mechanism to ensure that the plant will be able to spread its seed. If you get dried goldenrod flowers in the store, they will often look like white fluff with seeds rather than the golden flowers that they should be.

When you get your goldenrod flowers home, leave the bag on its side to allow insects a chance to crawl out. There are some tiny bugs that love to hide among the flower clusters.

Goldenrod leaves can be harvested in early summer before the plant flowers, when they are most tender and aromatic. Harvest the entire leafy stalk.

Harvesting goldenrod flowering tops in the Cascades in mid-August

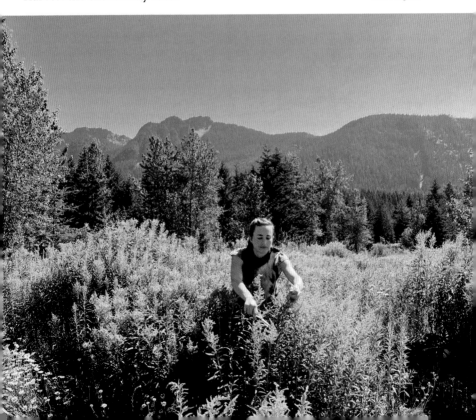

As with other roots, harvest goldenrod root in the spring or fall when the plant is more dormant. Use a digging fork to loosen the soil around the crown of the plant and carefully unearth the root. You will need to brush and pick soil out and then take it home and spray it down with a hose before scrubbing thoroughly with a brush. Note that harvesting the root kills the plant, so please harvest from a dense patch and be mindful about how much you are taking. If you are lucky enough to come upon some that needs to be salvaged, even better!

Goldenrod is a great plant to introduce into your garden by digging up a little start in the wild with some soil, putting it into a little pot, and bringing it home. Let it sit in the pot for a few days before putting it in the ground.

Medicinal Uses of Goldenrod

Goldenrod flower is warming, sweet, and aromatic, with an organ affinity for the kidneys, lungs, and stomach. It is diuretic, gently expectorant, antihistamine, anti-inflammatory to the lungs, and warming to the stomach and bowels.

I see it most often used in teas and tinctures for hay fever and other allergies. The aerial parts of goldenrod contain large

BRUISE LINIMENT   *Makes 1 ounce*

A liniment is basically a tincture that is exclusively for topical use, especially for musculoskeletal pain and injuries. For this liniment, you can make your own goldenrod and St. John's wort tinctures, or use store-bought tinctures. Take care not to get the liniment on clothing, as it can stain.

Dosage: Spray on bruised area several times a day, rubbing in vigorously with your hand.

---

1 tablespoon goldenrod leaf or flower tincture (see Tincture Ratio Chart)
1 tablespoon St. John's wort flower tincture (see Tincture Ratio Chart)

Pour both tinctures into a 1-ounce amber spray bottle using a small funnel. Strain well first if there are bits, as they will get caught in the spraying mechanism and clog it.
The liniment will keep for up to 5 years.

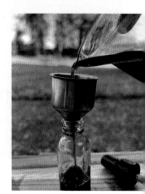

HAY FEVER TEA FORMULA   *Makes 1.5 ounces*

Drink this classic tea formula throughout allergy season. It is particularly good for inflamed sinuses and runny nose. If you are using wildcrafted plant material that you have dried yourself, you will need to garble the herbs first (pull the flowers and leaves off the stems and discard the stems) and break up larger pieces to make them easier to mix together. Carefully measure the herbs with a kitchen scale.

Dosage: Use 1 to 2 tablespoons per cup. Infuse for 10 minutes, covered. Drink 1 to 2 cups per day.

0.5 ounce dried goldenrod flower
0.5 ounce dried elderflower
0.5 ounce dried nettle leaf

Combine all three herbs in a medium bowl. With your hands, massage the herbs together, removing any residual stems and breaking up larger pieces.
Store in a 16-ounce jar in a cool, dark place for up to 1 year.

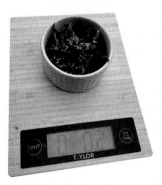 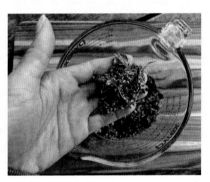

amounts of quercetin, which is an anti-inflammatory that helps curb histamine reactions. Goldenrod flower is classically combined with elderflower—they taste pretty good together in tea with a little honey.

Goldenrod can be used for problems of the kidneys and bladder, such as urinary tract infections (though not as a primary herb for this), gout, weak bladder, and mild edema (water retention in the feet and ankles).

Goldenrod leaf was once used in Europe as a vulnerary (topical-wound healer), much like we use plantain leaf in modern herbalism. You can make and apply the infused oil, wash the affected area with tea, or chew the leaves a bit and apply that topically as a poultice. It can be used for bruising and contusion-type injuries as well. Arnica, the most popular plant for bruising and swelling, is more difficult to find and not as sheerly abundant as goldenrod. I think we should revive the use of goldenrod for this purpose!

My friend Natasha Clarke turned me on to using the root of goldenrod, which is even more aromatic than the flowers. Several years ago, I ran into a goldenrod patch that had been dug up by a bulldozer, so I grabbed the roots from the mountain of dirt and made a tincture. The tincture of the root is sweeter and more aromatic than the flowers—flavors that would suggest its use as an expectorant and lung tonic.

Making Medicine with Goldenrod

The most commonly used preparation of goldenrod is a hot infusion of the dried flowers. You can also make a tincture of the fresh flowering tops (see Tincture Ratio Chart). I like to remove the thicker stems before tincturing, and I typically include some leaves as well. Puree the flowers with the alcohol in a blender to increase potency. Use the tincture in combination with St. John's wort tincture to treat bruises (see Bruise Liniment).

Cautions

Because goldenrod is a diuretic, avoid taking it with pharmaceutical diuretic medications.

Gumweed

Grindelia integrifolia
Asteraceae (sunflower family)

Puget Sound gumweed (*Grindelia integrifolia*) is the most common species of gumweed in the Pacific Northwest and grows almost exclusively on the coastline around the Puget Sound. You can collect seeds and plant it elsewhere, but in the wild it sticks to the edge of the tidal zone. There are several other Puget Sound coastline specialists that are beach dwellers, like silver beachweed (*Ambrosia chamissonis*) and American searocket (*Cakile edentula*). No matter where you are in the world, coastlines will always have a set of specialists that are uniquely adapted to the harsh, salty environment.

There is also another species of *Grindelia* that grows east of the Cascades: curlycup gumweed (*Grindelia squarrosa*). I have never seen it myself, so my experience is limited to my local species. However, curlycup is the most common gumweed in the United States, and many herbalists use that species. As far as I know, they have identical medicinal uses.

Harvesting Gumweed

Harvest the resinous buds of gumweed just before they open, when the resin is visible on the top of the bud. You can pluck off the buds with your fingernail or use scissors. A parchmentpaper bag is recommended for harvest as the resin will stick to most other things. Gumweed blooms in July and August, so the

LEFT A gumweed bud with visible resin **RIGHT** Puget Sound gumweed growing in the San Juan Islands alongside yarrow and coastal mugwort

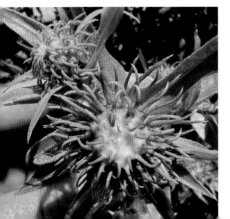
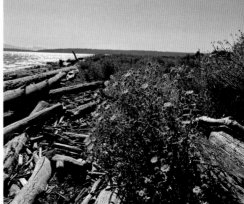

best harvests are earlier in the season. Like calendula, when you harvest the flowers, the plant generates more in its place.

Seeds can be collected from late August to November. I have had a lot of luck harvesting wild seeds, germinating them, and turning them into beautiful garden plants that are very drought tolerant. I strongly recommend cultivating gumweed so that we don't pressure the wild stock, given that gumweed's preferred habitat has been heavily impacted by coastline development. That said, the harvest of gumweed is relatively low impact as long as you leave some flowers on the plant for pollinators to visit.

Medicinal Uses of Gumweed

Harvesting gumweed buds along a beach on the Puget Sound

Gumweed presents an excellent example of the "doctrine of signatures," a concept dating back to the ancient Greeks that says plants have visible characteristics that resemble the illnesses they cure. In the case of gumweed, the sticky resin that covers the buds resembles phlegm, and gumweed is primarily used as an expectorant for dislodging it.

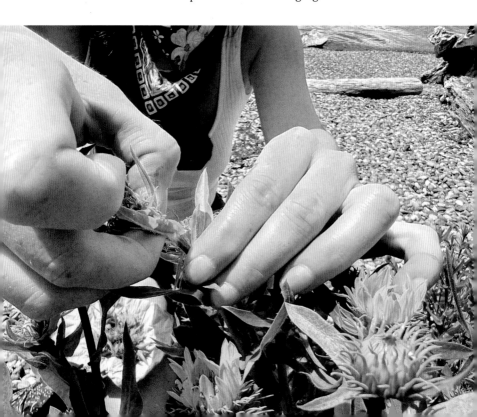

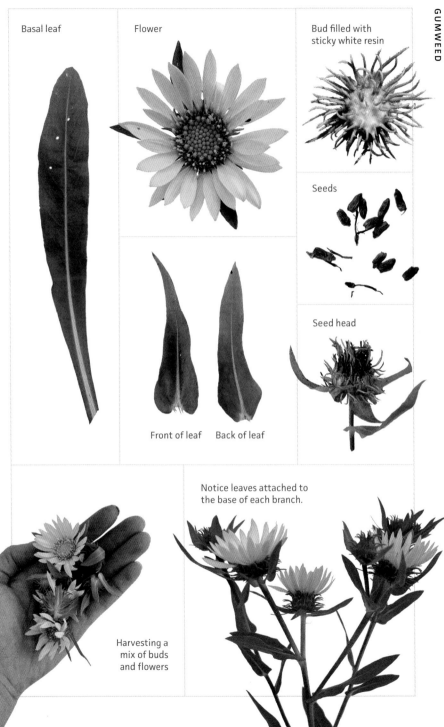

Basal leaf

Flower

Bud filled with sticky white resin

Seeds

Seed head

Front of leaf   Back of leaf

Notice leaves attached to the base of each branch.

Harvesting a mix of buds and flowers

Gumweed is irritating and opening in nature, stirring up stubborn phlegm and helping to move it out. Use gumweed buds when you can feel the phlegm rattling around in your lungs but your cough is not productive. Your throat might feel a bit dry, and the cough might be a bit spasmodic. It can also be used for dry sinus conditions with a phlegm component.

FRESH GUMWEED FOLK TINCTURE
Makes about 4 ounces

Gumweed tincture is the preparation I use most often. Given the strength of the herb, gumweed tincture is taken in smaller doses than other tinctures. I take a few drops at a time for stuck, phlegmy coughs and asthma with rattling phlegm in the lungs. It is important in this recipe to use high-proof alcohol because resins are soluble in alcohol but not water. You can water it down just a bit if the alcohol is too harsh, but use no more than 1 tablespoon of water as you don't want to dilute the medicine too much.

Dosage: Take 3 to 5 drops every 1 to 2 hours for acute cough; take no more than 10 drops in one dose.

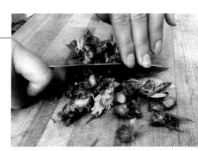

1 cup fresh gumweed buds
4 to 6 fluid ounces of 75 percent alcohol
    (mix 3 parts 190-proof alcohol and
    1 part water to achieve this)

Chop the buds carefully with a knife. They are quite sticky, so you will likely need to clean the knife and your hands with alcohol afterward to remove the resin.
    Put the buds into a clean 8-ounce jar, packing loosely.

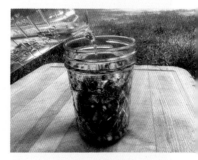

    Pour alcohol over the buds until it just covers them.
    Seal the jar with the lid and label well.
    Let sit in a cool, dark place. You can check your tincture after 24 hours of steeping to see its color change; it should be bright green! The color will fade with time. Leave it to macerate for 4 weeks, shaking occasionally.
    Strain through cheesecloth or a fine-mesh strainer. Since the buds contain a lot of resin, there is a chance that they will leave a sticky residue on any equipment you use.
    Store in an 8-ounce jar for no more than 5 years.

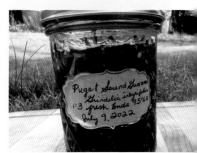

Similarly, gumweed is used for asthma when mucus obstructs the bronchioles and creates difficulty breathing. It's used for chronic bronchitis as well.

I typically use it in a formula with other herbs, making gumweed about 10 percent of the final product. Using stronger herbs like gumweed in small amounts in formulas is one way to ensure you're taking a small dose.

Making Medicine with Gumweed

The resins in gumweed are alcohol soluble and hydrophobic, which means that a higher percentage of alcohol is best to make a tincture. I typically end up making a folk tincture of the buds, which means that I don't measure. The tincture turns bright green in the middle of its maceration period—a fun, sciencey delight that's in store for you (see the recipe for Fresh Gumweed Folk Tincture).

A decoction of gumweed buds has been used in the past, though that preparation is out of favor now. In my experience, the buds are really hard to dry and store, which is why I don't prepare them that way. Low and slow heat can eventually extract resin into water though, so try a decoction if you feel the desire to do so!

Gumweed does not taste great, so my friend Kate makes a lovely infused honey with fresh buds, and an elixir (soaked in alcohol and honey), both of which are delicious and effective. I might recommend a less offensive expectorant—such as mullein, goldenrod, or thyme—if the specific powers of gumweed are not needed.

Cautions

Gumweed irritates the kidneys in large doses and should be taken only in small doses for short periods of time.

Hawthorn

Crataegus monogyna, C. douglasii
Rosaceae (rose family)

The one-seed hawthorn (*Crataegus monogyna*) originally came from Europe and is an important part of many herbal traditions. It was brought to Oregon around the year 1800 and has spread all over the Pacific Northwest since then. It has strong associations with May Day and fertility in the British Isles, and there is much folklore surrounding it.

One-seed hawthorn is the most common species of hawthorn in the Pacific Northwest, but not the only one. According to the Biota of North America Program, there are 153 species of *Crataegus* in the US. Washington alone has thirteen naturalized species. You can tell that you have one-seed hawthorn quite easily because, as the name implies, the red fruits will have one seed rather than two or more. Our other common local species is the native black hawthorn (*Crataegus douglasii*), named for the black color of its berries.

One-seed hawthorn is considered invasive in the city of Seattle and other places throughout the country. It is indeed rather enthusiastic in its growth and difficult to remove; if you cut it down, it often sprouts right back up from the stump. Because these trees are so hard to kill by simply cutting them down, the city gets rid of them by installing bullet-like herbicide plugs that inject poison into the tree and root system.

One-seed hawthorn received its invasive status because it grows in fields—birds eat the berries and then poop the seeds out miles away—and blocks the movement of livestock in their grazing pastures.

Although flowers are typically white, some one-seed hawthorn flowers are pink! Those are still the same species but a different phenotype. The flowers and young leaves are edible and can be put in salads.

Some of these flowers have released pollen (black stamens), and some haven't (pink stamens).

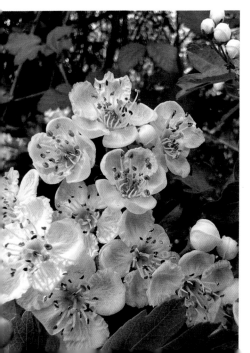

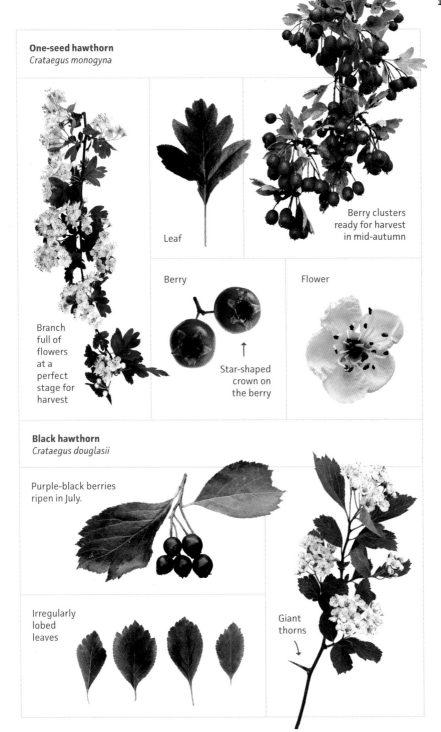

One-seed hawthorn
Crataegus monogyna

Leaf

Berry clusters ready for harvest in mid-autumn

Branch full of flowers at a perfect stage for harvest

Berry

Star-shaped crown on the berry

Flower

Black hawthorn
Crataegus douglasii

Purple-black berries ripen in July.

Irregularly lobed leaves

Giant thorns

Harvesting Hawthorn

Hawthorn typically blooms in May, or late April in the southern areas of our region. The trees all bloom at roughly the same time in a given area, and blooms last for about a week before the flowers are spent and the petals fall. The flowers should be harvested as soon as they open, with some still in bud if possible. It is better to harvest flowers that have pink stamens rather than black. The pink means that the pollen has not yet been released and the flower is still young. As soon as the pollen is released, the stamens turn black and the flower starts to lose its constituents.

Hawthorn flowers smell like rotting corpses—and indeed share similar chemistry—in order to attract pollinators. Sometimes if you are walking by a patch on a May day and the wind is blowing in the right direction, you will get a grand whiff of it! This means that hawthorn medicine—especially the tea—can have a bit of a funky taste that some folks don't care for.

I harvest the berries in October, though some people harvest as early as late September and as late as November. The trick is to get them while they have a lot of their sugars and less of the sour and astringent compounds that will be present if you harvest too early. I test the berries for ripeness by squishing them: the flesh should be soft and a bit orange-yellow rather than white. Another way to check is to taste them to see if they are starting to get a bit sweet, which is what you want. If you wait to harvest too late, the berries begin to mold—indicated by black on the surface.

Harvesting hawthorn berries with friends

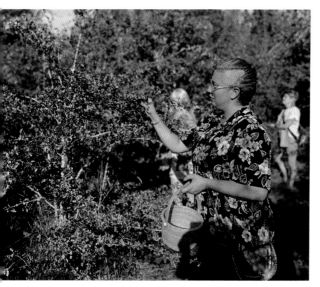

Our native black hawthorn is a little more elusive than the enthusiastic and non-native one-seed hawthorn. Black hawthorn berries ripen much earlier, in July and August, and are dark black in color. Because they are rarer and have fewer berries, I mostly leave them for the birds unless I find a really good group of trees.

Medicinal Uses of Hawthorn

Hawthorn is first and foremost a medicine for the heart and blood vessels. It strengthens the vessel walls and the heart muscle, lending itself well to irregular heartbeats, cardiac insufficiency, atherosclerosis, and a host of other heart-related illnesses. Like most strengthening medicines, it works slowly over time and works best as a preventative, so make it part of a daily routine in whatever way you can.

Hawthorn leaf and flower are often used for poor peripheral circulation as they help strengthen and smooth blood vessel

---

IN-FIELD TINCTURE OF HAWTHORN FLOWER   *Makes about 8 ounces*

Making a tincture out in the field captures the plant at its freshest and makes the project feel more special, infused with the energy of the experience. This recipe features hawthorn flowers—as many as you can fit in whatever jar you bring along with you—and uses the folk method rather than the standardized method for tincturing. You can cut the flowers into smaller pieces directly into the jar with scissors. Scale this recipe up or down depending on your need. I often make a 32-ounce jar, especially if I plan on sharing the tincture with friends and family.

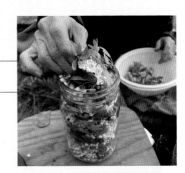

Dosage: Take 30 to 60 drops 2 to 3 times a day.

---

2 cups freshly harvested hawthorn flowers
About 1 cup 100-proof alcohol (50 percent),
    such as vodka, plus more as needed

Cut the hawthorn flowers into smaller pieces with a knife or a pair of scissors, filling a 16-ounce jar. Tamp them lightly with your fingers.

Pour alcohol into the jar until it reaches the level of the flowers. Add more alcohol if needed to cover properly.

Seal the jar with the lid and label well.

Let sit in a cool, dark place for 1 month, shaking occasionally. Strain through cheesecloth and store in the same jar for up to 5 years.

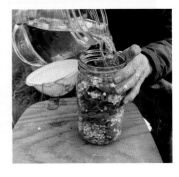

walls, creating less friction in the system, which can slow the blood down. For this same reason, hawthorn can be used for high blood pressure, especially when inflammation is the cause.

Atherosclerosis is the buildup of plaque on damaged areas of the blood vessel walls, which can eventually lead to a heart attack. Because of hawthorn's anti-inflammatory and antioxidant compounds, hawthorn can reduce the "sticky" places on the vessel walls where plaque accumulates. This remedy is best used as a preventative for anyone who has atherosclerosis.

Anxiety and grief that involve a closing of the heart and heaviness in the chest are good indications for hawthorn. I have had students report, after a few weeks of experimenting with hawthorn, that they cried a bunch and felt much lighter afterward.

Hawthorn can also be used in formulas for allergies because of its anti-inflammatory effects, along with herbs like elderflower and goldenrod.

Making Medicine with Hawthorn

Hawthorn leaf and flower are best as a tea or tincture (see Tincture Ratio Chart and In-Field Tincture of Hawthorn Flower). In tea, I mix them with hibiscus for blood vessel health, with lemon balm and tulsi for anxiety, and with cinnamon and rosemary for circulation.

Hawthorn berries can be made into a decoction or a tincture (see Tincture Ratio Chart). The fresh berries have a lot of pectin in them, which is what gels jam, so sometimes the tincture will turn out thick and gloppy. I have noticed that this happens especially if you harvest the berries too early. Because the gloppy texture can make the tincture difficult to strain and clog the glass droppers used to dose tinctures, some people prefer to make their tinctures from dried berries to avoid the problem altogether.

My students especially enjoy making an oxymel with fresh hawthorn berries, which turns out thicker than oxymels made with other plants and is more like a sauce or jam. There are also a lot of exciting condiments you can make with the berries. I have made delicious chutney, jam, jelly, cordial, and fruit leather (see Hawthorn Chutney). The trick is to use a food mill to remove the seeds.

HAWTHORN CHUTNEY

Makes about 4 cups

This recipe comes from Suzanne Tabert, the founder and student mentor at the Cedar Mountain Herb School (cedarmountainherbs.com) in Seattle and Sandpoint, Idaho, as well as adjunct faculty at Bastyr University. I've been making it for years and love eating it with roasted meat in the wintertime. It makes a great replacement for cranberry sauce. A food mill is a key part of this recipe as removing hawthorn seeds can be difficult otherwise. If you don't have a food mill, use the back of a spoon to push the mixture through a mesh strainer, but know that this method is a challenge. Be sure to remove any leaves from the hawthorn sprigs, but stems are okay.

4½ pounds hawthorn berries
1 quart apple cider vinegar
2 tablespoons sea or mineral salt
A few sprigs of fresh thyme
3 cups organic light-brown sugar
2 tablespoons ground ginger
1 tablespoon ground nutmeg
½ tablespoon ground cloves
½ tablespoon ground allspice
½ teaspoon ground black pepper

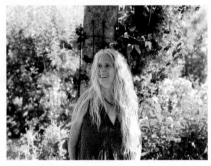

Suzanne Tabert

Put the berries in a 6-quart pot, add the vinegar and salt, and bring to a boil. Once boiling, turn down the heat to a simmer, cover the pot, and cook the berries until soft—about 45 minutes.

Pass the cooked hawthorn berries through a food mill to remove the seeds. If the berries are still hot, be careful of the steam. The hawthorn paste will come out of the bottom. You should end up with 2 pints of pulp. This takes patience. Put on some good music.

Rinse out the 6-quart pot and spoon the hawthorn paste back into it. Remove the leaves from the sprigs of thyme and add to the pot along with the sugar and spices.

Cook for 10 minutes on medium heat until the sugar is completely melted and the paste is hot all the way through. Stir constantly to keep the sugar from scorching.

Store the hawthorn chutney in a sealed container in the fridge for immediate use and use within 30 days, or until signs of mold appear. Alternatively, spoon the hawthorn berry chutney into plastic freezer jars and freeze for up to 6 months. The chutney can also be canned using a water bath if you're familiar with that technique.

Horsetail

Equisetum telmateia, E. arvense, E. hyemale
Equisetaceae (horsetail family)

You will find horsetail growing in ditches, ponds, near creeks, and in wet areas on hillsides. Wherever you see horsetail, be assured there is some source of water there, even if the ground looks fairly dry.

Horsetail is not a flowering or seeding plant. It reproduces with spores, which are released by the fertile shoots in the spring (see photos). The spores are green and powdery. Water carries the spores to form new colonies, much like the way in which mushrooms and mosses reproduce. The vegetative shoots, which are green and shaped like a bottle brush, come out immediately after the spores are released. They are for photosynthesizing and creating energy for the plant and are not involved in reproduction.

Horsetail roots grow extremely deep, which is how this 230-million-year-old plant was able to survive two major extinction events. Its ecological role is to pull minerals from deep within the earth up to the surface. Rain washes away soil minerals over time, so those minerals have to be continually replenished.

LEFT Fertile shoots of giant horsetail coming up in early spring **RIGHT** A cluster of giant horsetail vegetative shoots

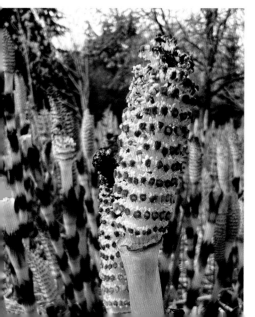
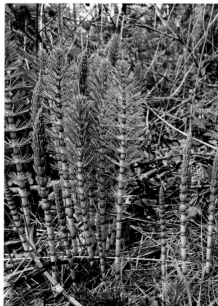

Giant horsetail *Equisetum telmateia*		Scouring rush *Equisetum hyemale*	Common horsetail *Equisetum arvense*
Fertile shoot, about to release its spores	Vegetative shoot	Combined fertile and vegetative shoot	Shoot harvest
			Vegetative shoot

Harvesting Horsetail

We have three main species in our bioregion: giant horsetail (*Equisetum telmateia*), common horsetail (*Equisetum arvense*), and scouring rush (*Equisetum hyemale*). My favorite to harvest is giant horsetail.

Harvest the vegetative, green shoots of horsetail in April and May. The general consensus is to harvest before the arms have dropped below 90 degrees as it then loses its potency. Use clippers to snip off newer shoots, and put your harvest in a paper bag or basket. Horsetail shoots contain water in the stem, so although they dry quickly, they are at risk for mold. Avoid harvesting on wet or dewy days, and be sure to use your dehydrator to prevent mold if they're damp. Once dry, break them up with your hands and store in a paper bag or a jar.

Because of its affinity for groundwater, you want to be careful not to harvest horsetail in places where the water might be contaminated with heavy metals, human waste, or chemicals.

There's no need to worry about overharvesting any of the horsetail species. Because of the deep roots and the aggressive habit of the plant, it is actually quite hard to get rid of once it has established itself. Horsetail has been rather vilified because livestock can get sick if they eat too much for too long. There are articles all over the internet on how to get it out of your

LEFT Harvesting common horsetail in sandy soil near the Puget Sound **RIGHT** I like to select newer shoots and clip them at the base. (Photo by Wren Morrow)

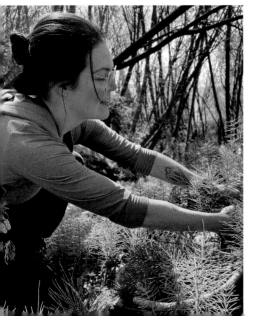
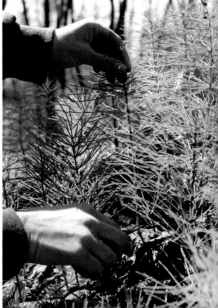

STRENGTHENING HAIR RINSE   *Makes 2 to 4 applications (about 1 quart)*

This hair-invigorating rinse is a slice of history. Nettle hair rinses have been used for centuries in various cultures to thicken and darken hair.

1 cup dried nettle leaf (broken up or chopped)
1 cup dried horsetail shoots (broken up or chopped)
Boiling water

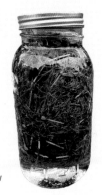

Put the nettles and horsetail in a quart-size jar and fill the jar with boiling water. Cover the jar with the lid and let sit for at least 1 hour. If you'd like some *really* potent stuff, let it sit overnight. Strain through a fine-mesh strainer and then pour it back into the jar to store.

Use up to half the tea to rinse your clean hair (can be applied to wet or dry hair), focusing on rubbing it into the scalp. Don't rinse with water, but let your hair dry with the tea in it. Use the remaining tea over the next few days, storing no longer than 4 days.

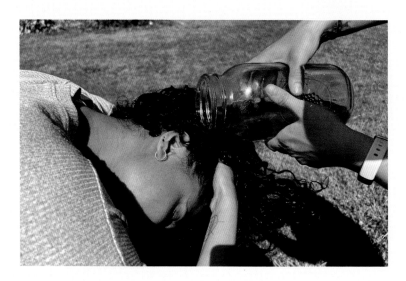

pasture or garden. Many warn that it is very difficult to eradicate, as even herbicides rarely can kill it. But unlike other aggressive weeds, horsetail doesn't outcompete other plants, so as a gardener, I would accept its presence in my garden and use it for medicine and food.

Medicinal Uses of Horsetail

Horsetail is one of the best sources of water-soluble silica. Silica increases the uptake of calcium and encourages the formation of collagen, both of which help bone, teeth, hair, and nails. Not only does horsetail have a history of use for bone strengthening, it has also been studied for its use in preventing and treating osteoporosis with good results. We herbalists use horsetail tea as a strengthening hair rinse (see recipe) or nail bath, or we drink it as a hot infusion to strengthen all the aforementioned structures.

Horsetail is also a diuretic and an important herb for strengthening the bladder. You can add it to teas for these purposes (see Bladder-Strengthening Tea Formula) as well as for urinary tract infections. Horsetail is used in formulas for interstitial cystitis and incontinence.

The tea is also high in quercetin, which can help reduce allergic responses and inflammation. You can combine it in a tea blend with other quercetin-rich plants, like goldenrod, elderflower, and nettle, and drink it throughout allergy season.

BLADDER-STRENGTHENING
TEA FORMULA

Makes 1.1 ounces loose-leaf tea (about 1 cup)

This tea formula is for folks with frequent urination, frequent UTIs, bladder irritations, or a weak bladder. It is astringent, cooling, diuretic, and soothing. Any herbs needed for this recipe that you do not harvest yourself can be purchased online (see Resources). Try to avoid drinking the tea right before bed, as you will need to get up to pee in the night.

Dosage: Use 1 to 2 tablespoons per cup. Infuse for 10 minutes, covered. Drink 1 to 2 cups per day.

0.5 ounce dried marshmallow root
0.2 ounce dried horsetail shoots
0.2 ounce dried agrimony leaf
0.2 ounce dried goldenrod flowers

Combine all ingredients in a medium bowl. Mix well.
Store in a jar for up to 3 years.

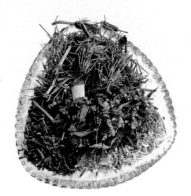

Making Medicine with Horsetail

A hot infusion of horsetail shoots works quite well and tastes fairly neutral. If you are looking for a particularly powerful extraction of the minerals, try decocting it on the stove, or add a dash of vinegar to the tea water.

Because acidic solutions extract minerals incredibly well, horsetail infused vinegar is a nice mineral tonic. You can add other high-mineral herbs along with it, such as nettle, alfalfa, and chickweed.

Horsetail tincture is made only from the dry plant material (see Tincture Ratio Chart), though the tincture is rarely used medicinally.

Cautions

The vegetative shoots of horsetail should not be eaten raw. They contain an enzyme called thiaminase that breaks down thiamine (B_1), but fortunately, the enzyme is naturally destroyed in the drying process. In large amounts, thiaminase could cause serious health complications, such as blindness and paralysis. However, it is unlikely a human would eat enough to cause complications that serious; it is more of a danger to cows, horses, and other animals.

Mugwort

Artemisia suksdorfii, *A.* spp.
Asteraceae (sunflower family)

We have many species of mugwort in the Pacific Northwest, all with lobed leaves, silver undersides, and a funky, aromatic smell. My favorite of them all—and also the most common—is coastal mugwort. It grows mostly around the Puget Sound and along the Pacific coast on rocky hillsides. However, this plant is not limited to the coastline, despite what its name may suggest. You can also find it growing farther inland on rocky hillsides and sometimes even up in the mountains. My favorite patch of coastal mugwort is in the Cascades at around 3,000 feet in elevation, where it grows on an exposed mountain slope alongside oxeye daisy and goldenrod.

The name mugwort may come from its use in beer making. Before hops were used universally, many other herbs were used in the brewing process, including mugwort. One of my students gave a delightful presentation on this plant and made a delicious mugwort ale for the occasion.

LEFT Coastal mugwort just beginning to bud along a forest service road in the Cascades
RIGHT Coastal mugwort in flower

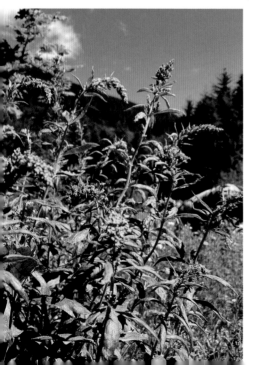
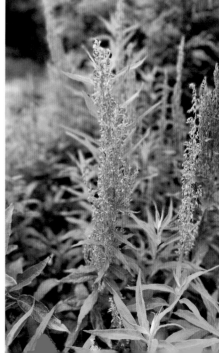

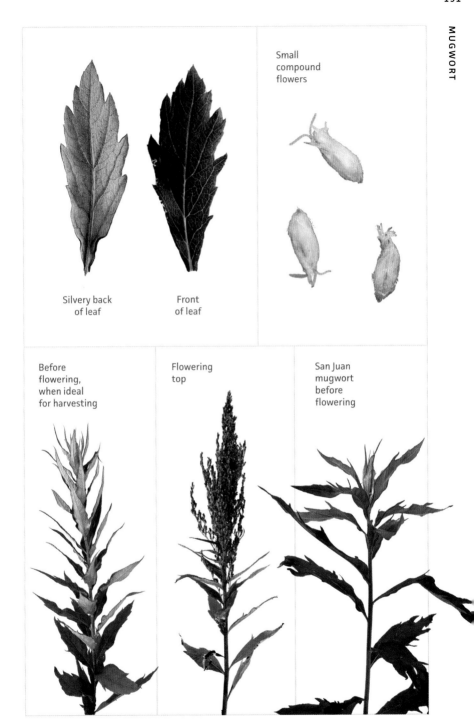

Silvery back
of leaf

Front
of leaf

Small
compound
flowers

Before
flowering,
when ideal
for harvesting

Flowering
top

San Juan
mugwort
before
flowering

Harvesting Mugwort

Coastal mugwort has a distinct aromatic smell, so check your ID with a sniff. Goldenrod, a close look-alike, does not smell as aromatic and also does not have leaves with silver-haired undersides like mugwort.

Harvest the leafy tops of mugwort before it flowers, typically in early June and extending into July and maybe August. By August, most stalks will have flowers that are browning and turning to seed; while the seeds are nicely aromatic, they are not as nice as the leaves. Clip the top two-thirds of the stalk, which has the healthiest-looking leaves. The nodes of the remaining leaves will sprout new shoots from the sides, much like nettle.

Note your harvest spot, as mugwort is a perennial and will come back year after year in the same spot. Skip a year or two if you notice it getting smaller, though. Mugwort is fairly abundant where it grows but could easily suffer from overharvesting due to its popularity.

Coastal mugwort grows vigorously in a garden, so you could introduce this native plant to a dry, sunny spot in your yard. Either collect the ultra-tiny seeds in the fall and start your own,

Clip the top two-thirds of coastal mugwort stalks.

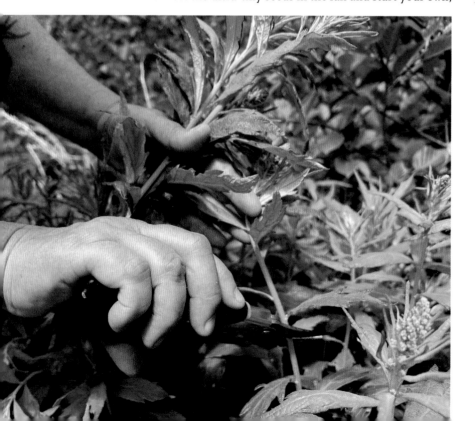

buy a start from a local medicinal herb grower, or dig up a tiny start from the wild that's in a spot where it will perish anyway. Mugwort will grow in a pot and might actually yield enough for harvest if you give it a really large pot and plenty of care.

Medicinal Uses of Mugwort

Mugwort is perhaps most famous for its use in enhancing dreams. I have heard mixed reviews—some claim they have had wild dreams and will never use it again because it was too intense, some love it, and some see no effect at all. This just goes to show that everyone has their own unique experience with each plant. I encourage you to try it out for yourself. For this use, you can put the leaf under your pillow, drink a tea of it before bed, take a tincture, or even smoke it as an herbal cigarette.

One of the first things you will notice upon tasting mugwort is its bitterness. This, of course, indicates its use as a bitter, which means that it stimulates secretions from the liver and can be used for digestion. But this is not a common use for mugwort as there are better and tastier plants for the job, like chamomile.

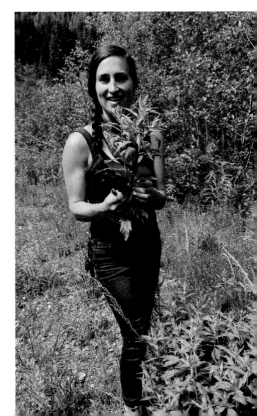

Harvesting mugwort among slide alders along a forest service road in the Cascades

Across cultures who use mugwort, almost all of them use it for women's health. Mugwort has an emmenagogue action, which means it can bring on a missed or absent period. Mugwort is also used for certain menstrual conditions because it warms the uterus and moves stagnant blood. Keep in mind that it may be too stimulating and warming for some people, so carefully note your reaction and stop taking it if it seems to be causing more pain or bleeding.

Korean women's bathhouses often have a tub of mugwort tea to pour on yourself. These mugwort baths are meant to keep skin young and healthy. Mugwort helps oily and acne-prone skin with its anti-inflammatory and antimicrobial properties. It protects your skin from free-radical damage because of its antioxidant actions.

SELF-BURNING INCENSE

Makes ¼ to ½ cup

This recipe was inspired by Karica Laine, one of my first yearlong students. Years later she taught me how to make this incense. The recipe combines the flammable fuzz of mugwort with slow-burning tree resin, creating a loose incense that keeps itself lit. It is quite magical! Make it with copal, pine resin, myrrh, or frankincense. These resins can be purchased in bulk at some herb stores and online (see Resources). The resin must be very dry and hard in order to grind properly. If you are having trouble, try putting it in the freezer for a few hours. Sometimes pine resins are soft when you harvest, which would not work in this recipe. Be sure to remove the stems from the mugwort leaves before weighing.

0.3 ounce dried mugwort
   leaves with stems removed
0.4 ounce frankincense (or
   other resin)

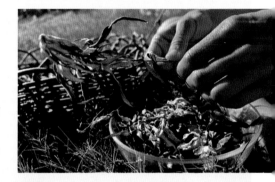

Put the mugwort leaves into your herb grinder, being careful not to pack too tightly so the grinder can still work. Grind until it is a nice fuzz (see photos). You may need to shake the grinder.

Transfer the mugwort fuzz to a small bowl and add the resin to the grinder. Grind into a powder.

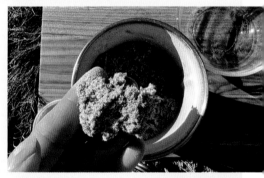

Put the mugwort back into the grinder with the resin and grind the two together, shaking well.

Pour into a small jar and store for up to 3 years.

To light, take a marble-size amount and put it on a rock or in a fire-safe bowl. Use your fingers to shape it into a pyramid. Use a lighter or match to light the top on fire. Let it burn for a few seconds, then blow it out to leave an ember. Keep blowing for a few seconds to build the ember. Don't leave unattended!

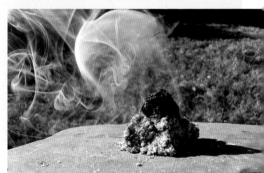

Making Medicine with Mugwort

A hot infusion of mugwort makes a great bath or hair rinse but does not make a tasty tea given its bitterness. Some people put mugwort in tea formulas, though, so experiment!

Mugwort alcohol intermediary oil is wonderfully aromatic and a deep green (to make your own, use the Bleeding Heart Alcohol Intermediary Oil recipe, replacing bleeding heart with mugwort). I love to infuse it in almond or apricot seed oil and use it as a face oil. Mugwort helps prevent wrinkles and repairs aging skin. Mugwort hydrosol is also lovely on the skin (see the Wild Carrot Hydrosol recipe for instructions on how to make a hydrosol at home).

You can make a tincture of fresh or dried mugwort leaf (see Tincture Ratio Chart).

When you grind the dried leaves or rub them in your hands, they become a fuzzy mass that resembles pillow stuffing. This fuzzy material burns well and can be used for herbal cigarettes, incense (see recipe), and moxibustion, a traditional Chinese therapy.

Cautions

Mugwort is not safe to consume during pregnancy.

Mullein

Verbascum thapsus
Scrophulariaceae (figwort family)

Great mullein (*Verbascum thapsus*) was introduced to the United States from Europe so that its seeds could be used to stun fish and make them easier to catch—a method that is now illegal. It now grows in almost all areas of the country and is considered a noxious weed in some places. It can survive in dry wasteland-type soils and even gravel, making it a great weed. What's more, the seeds of mullein can remain viable in the soil for hundreds of years! Though this may not delight the Department of Transportation, it certainly delights herbalists.

Mullein has a great affinity for burn sites, especially on the east side of the Cascades. You will find it mostly in dry, open areas. The grassy median strips in the middle of freeways and railroad tracks are places I've seen mullein thrive, which are both places I would not harvest because of pollution, unfortunately.

There are other species of mullein that grow in our area, but great mullein is the largest and most common.

LEFT Flowering mullein in a ponderosa pine forest east of the Cascades **RIGHT** A basal rosette from above. Avoid harvesting leaves when wet as they mold easily.

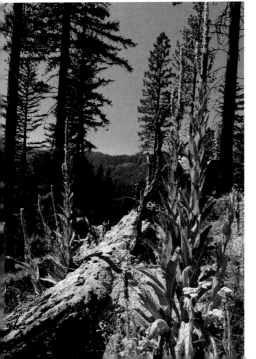
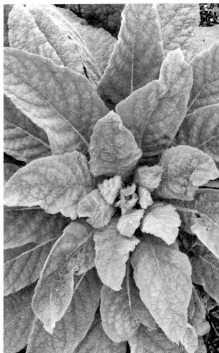

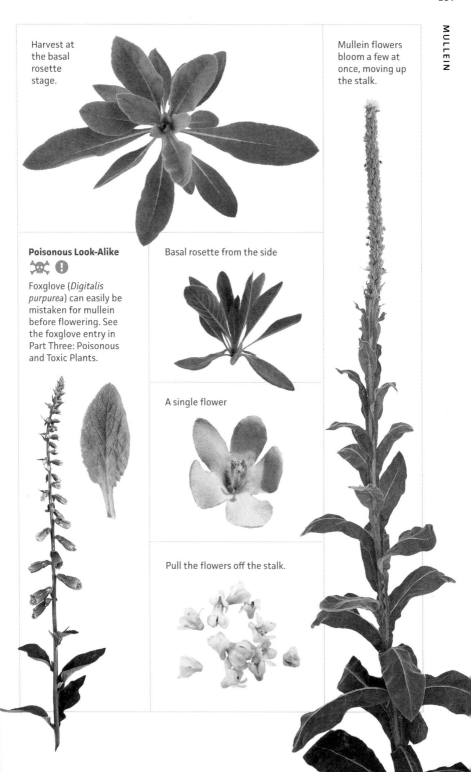

Harvest at the basal rosette stage.

Mullein flowers bloom a few at once, moving up the stalk.

Poisonous Look-Alike

Foxglove (*Digitalis purpurea*) can easily be mistaken for mullein before flowering. See the foxglove entry in Part Three: Poisonous and Toxic Plants.

Basal rosette from the side

A single flower

Pull the flowers off the stalk.

Harvesting Mullein

Mullein is a biennial, which means that in its first year it is just leaves. In the second year it shoots up an epic flower stalk, creates seeds, and disperses them; and then the whole plant dies in the fall of that year.

The ideal time to harvest mullein leaf is when the plant is in its vegetative state and has not yet started to climb into the air to flower. That means the fall of the first year or the spring of the second year are the best times. In a pinch, you can harvest the leaves from the flowering plant; they still have valuable medicine to offer.

The roots, too, can be harvested in the fall of the first year or spring of the second year. Do not harvest the roots once the flower stalk starts to appear, as the energy is no longer in the root. The taproot has fleshy bark and a very woody inner structure. You can use a digging fork to unearth it and then scrub it off with water. Because the leaves will come with it, it's nice to harvest the root and leaves at the same time.

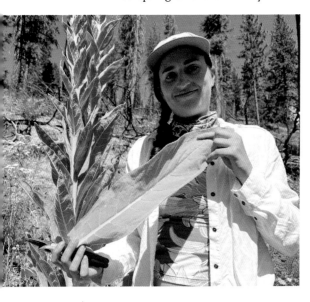

Harvesting mullein leaves in a ponderosa pine forest east of the Cascades

Each plant staggers its bloom times, so only a handful of plants in an area will be flowering at the same time. This means that flowers will need to be picked in batches. Sometimes you can get lucky and find a thick field of mullein in flower, which is the best opportunity to harvest the flowers.

It is incredibly easy to harvest mullein seeds—each plant has thousands of seeds. Just tip the seed stalk upside down, and the little brown seeds will fall out like sand. The seeds are rather tiny, so bring a small paper bag or a jar to store them in. You can help new patches form by spreading the seeds about, wielding the stalk like a magic wand. Spread them in the wild or your garden (but check local regulations first to ensure mullein isn't classified as a noxious weed in your area).

Medicinal Uses of Mullein

There are four different medicinal parts of mullein: leaves, flowers, roots, and seeds. The leaves are mucolytic, which means they help reduce the production of mucus. This makes them very helpful for phlegmy coughs, especially stuck ones. The leaves are also demulcent, or moistening and soothing, and thus useful for coughs that have an element of irritation or dryness. Mullein leaf is a great addition to a tea for chronic cough or a cold or for someone recovering from a cold, a smoker, or someone with asthma. You could also use mullein leaf in a throat spray for singers or for sore throats in general.

Mullein flowers are demulcent, anti-inflammatory, and anti-allergy. A classic remedy for ear infections is an infused oil of mullein flowers and garlic, which I used with success many times when I was younger and had many ear infections. The flowers are also very effective for allergies and asthmatic bronchitis when infused in honey. The honey could also be taken for hoarseness or sore throat.

The roots have gained popularity in recent years due to the teachings of herbalists such as Jim McDonald. Jim recommends it topically for spinal misalignment and spinal injury and internally for incontinence.

SOOTHING COUGH TEA
Makes 1.5 ounces loose-leaf tea

This tea is gently expectorant, soothing to inflamed tissues, and antispasmodic. It is for those coughs that keep you up at night, when you can't quite dislodge phlegm with the hacking cough.

Be sure to strain the tea with a fine-mesh strainer or several layers of cheesecloth to remove the mullein hairs, which can irritate the throat. If you are having trouble with this, you can buy disposable tea bags.

Dosage: Use 1 tablespoon per cup. Infuse for 10 minutes, covered. Drink 2 to 3 cups a day as symptoms persist.

0.5 ounce dried wild cherry bark
0.4 ounce dried marshmallow root
0.4 ounce dried thyme
0.2 ounce dried mullein leaves

Combine all ingredients in a bowl. Mix well. Store in a jar for up to 2 years.

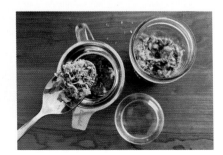

The seeds are sedative, which is the property that people as far back as the ancient Greeks utilized to catch fish. They crushed the seeds, tossed them in the water, and the fish would float to the top.

Making Medicine with Mullein

Mullein leaves should be dried before making medicine with them. The main two preparations I make are mullein leaf

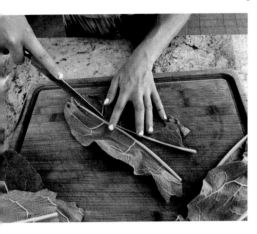

tincture (see Tincture Ratio Chart) and mullein leaf tea. Here are some ideas for making a tea formula: mullein leaf with marshmallow root for more demulcent action, with elecampane for a stronger expectorant action, with wild cherry bark for a spasmodic cough, or with thyme for a phlegmy and potentially infected cough (see Soothing Cough Tea). Take care to strain the tea well, as the little leaf hairs can irritate your throat as you drink.

Cut through the midrib to help the leaves dry faster and avoid mold.

Mullein flowers should be used fresh if possible. You can make an infused oil using the hot-water-bath method (see the instructions for Cottonwood Bud Infused Oil) or an infused honey (see Rose Infused Honey) also using a hot water bath. Don't turn the heat up too high on your hot water bath, as mullein flowers are delicate.

Mullein root can be tinctured fresh (see Tincture Ratio Chart) or made into an infused oil using the alcohol-intermediary-oil method or the hot-water-bath method.

Cautions

Strain mullein tea through a fine-mesh strainer or through cheesecloth in order to remove the small hairs. They're not necessarily harmful but can irritate the throat.

Nettle

Urtica dioica
Urticaceae (nettle family)

Stinging nettle gets a bad rap because of its stings, but it is actually one of the most useful plants in our bioregion. The leaves are edible; the seeds, roots, and leaves are medicinal; and the stems can be used to make textiles! Even its stings have been used medicinally in many different cultures for joint pain.

Nettle grows in patches and spreads by rhizome under the layer of dead leaves that always covers the soil in the Pacific Northwest. You might find it growing in a ravine in a city park, amid a patch of Himalayan blackberry, in a grove of alder trees next to your favorite hiking path, atop a city compost patch, or in a soggy meadow in the woods. What all of these places have in common are soft soil and plenty of water.

If you plan to introduce nettle into your yard, choose a spot that has partial shade and some sogginess, and throw down some dead leaves for its roots to spread under. You can dig rhizomes from the wild in February and replant them in your garden or grow them from seed. Or look for nettle plants at native plant sales.

The hairs in nettle are silicate vials filled with acids and neurochemicals—serotonin, epinephrine, and histamine—which break on contact and deposit their chemicals onto your skin, where they burn through the skin and rouse a local allergic response. It takes about five minutes for white welts to appear,

LEFT A thick patch of nettles at the edge of a forest in a local park **RIGHT** The tiny stinging hairs that cover nettle

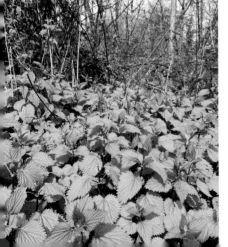
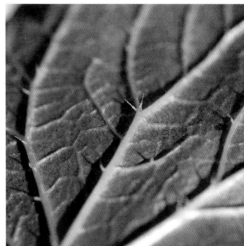

along with an interesting throbbing sensation from deeper in the skin, and later turn into a red itchy area that can last a few days. Nettle stings that affect areas with more nerves tend to be more annoying, such as on the pads of your fingers, under your fingernails, or in your mouth.

The best and easiest way to soothe a nettle sting is with a plantain leaf spit poultice. To make a spit poultice, take two to three leaves and chew them up into a rough pulp. Then take the wad of plantain leaf and press it on the affected area. Plantain likes to grow near trails where the soil is disturbed, so it will likely be nearby when you've been stung.

Harvesting Nettle

Nettle begins sprouting in February at lower elevations and in warm microclimates and can be ready for harvest mid-February. It can withstand a frost or two, and I have even seen it sprout through snow, though it won't really pick up its growth until after the last frost. In February, I look for nettles around the Puget Sound at sea level and in cities at low elevations. As you move into the foothills of the Cascades and other elevated places, the season starts in late March and is at its prime in April.

Nettle leaf should not be harvested for eating after it has flowered. One of my teachers, Cascade Anderson Geller, taught me not to harvest after it has grown past your knees. Also, harvest on a dry day so that you'll bring home dry nettles. Wet plants tend to mold. But if they are wet, use them immediately and don't try to dry or store them.

To harvest, you will need scissors, gloves, and a bag. Check for tiny green aphids before harvesting—some stands can really get infested in certain years. You can wash the aphids off if need be, but it's better to harvest those that have as few as possible. Grab hold of the nettle with your nondominant hand and, with the scissors in your dominant hand, snip the top of the stalk off, leaving at least two sets of leaves on the bottom.

Don't snip the plant at ground level, because then the nettle can't sprout back as easily. Two stems will grow up from where you cut, like when you snip the flowers off basil plants. Shake off any leaf debris or bugs, and drop it in your bag.

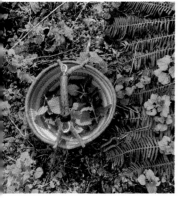

Nettles sprouting through sword fern fronds in March surround a basket of harvested leaves.

I harvest into a large paper grocery bag. When you get home, wear gloves and use tongs to pull them out of the bag for cooking and drying to avoid getting stung.

You will notice some nettle leaves are more purple or red than others, especially those that get more sunlight. Many plants produce anthocyanins and other leaf pigments to protect them from UV damage. These leaves are just as edible and medicinal!

Harvest nettle root in February or March, when the nettles are just sprouting up. Find the tiny nettle sprout and follow it down into the ground, where it will lead you to a rhizome. Gently tug the rhizomes out of the leaf duff, teasing out as much root as possible. I usually come up with foot-long sections of root. Take these home and wash them with water. Please harvest your nettle root only from particularly thick and abundant patches, as harvesting the roots has a much larger impact on the plant than harvesting the leaves.

Harvest nettle seed from June to August. Use gloves, as the stems that hold the seeds also have stinging hairs on them. Pluck the mature seed clusters off with your hands.

One caution I will say about harvesting nettles is that nettle is a bioaccumulator of minerals. This is great for calcium and iron, but if there is arsenic, mercury, or lead in the soil, the nettles will pick those up too. For this reason, avoid harvesting nettles next to old mines, busy roads, and in areas affected by industrial activity.

LEFT Snipping the top few sets of leaves from young nettles in April RIGHT The stinging hairs are most potent in the spring.

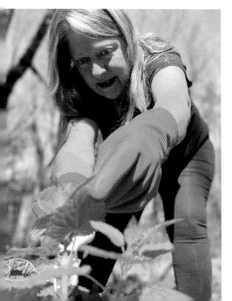
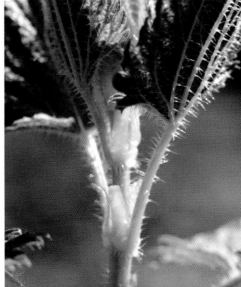

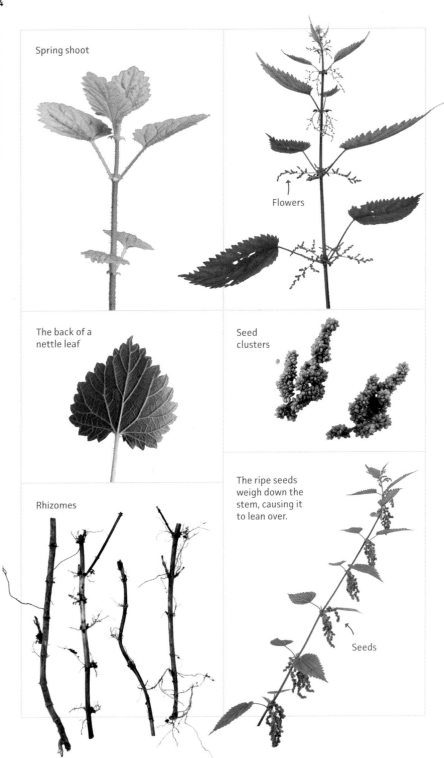

Spring shoot

Flowers

The back of a
nettle leaf

Seed
clusters

Rhizomes

The ripe seeds
weigh down the
stem, causing it
to lean over.

Seeds

Medicinal Uses of Nettle

All the parts of the nettle plant are medicinal and have slightly different uses, though the whole plant has some uniting characteristics. Its main organ affinity is the kidneys. All parts of the plant are also high in minerals, as nettle is a plant that accumulates minerals.

The most commonly used part of the plant is the leaf, which is most often employed for calming the allergic response, draining excess fluid, and providing minerals.

Nettle leaf is useful for hay fever, eczema, rashes, and even rheumatism. This action is attributed to the large amount of quercetin it contains, which is a compound that is anti-inflammatory and antihistamine. Horsetail, goldenrod, and elderflower also contain a lot of quercetin and are often combined with nettle in

---

NETTLE SEED SALT　　　　　　　　*Makes about 1 cup (2 spice shakers full)*

Nettle seed salt is a way to get small amounts of nettle seed in your diet. You can play around with what herbs to put into this mix, and you can even add toasted sesame seeds to create a more Japanese flavor. Use the salt to season soups, vegetables, or whatever strikes your fancy.

---

3 tablespoons dried nettle seeds
1 tablespoon dried oregano
1 tablespoon dried fennel seed
1 tablespoon dried thyme
1 tablespoon dried rosemary
½ cup sea salt

Put all the herbs in an herb grinder and grind together to produce a fine powder. Add the sea salt and grind. Grind more for a finer salt and less for a rougher salt. Store in a glass shaker and label well. The salt keeps for about a year.

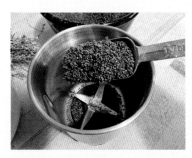
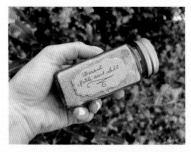

formula. Many of my students swear by nettle tea for preventing seasonal spring allergies. For this, they start drinking a few cups of tea per week in February at the beginning of pollen season and continue on through allergy season. Some folks argue that you need to use freeze-dried nettle leaf (which comes in capsules) for it to be effective, but plenty of people report great results using the tea.

Nettle is also a fairly strong diuretic. If you are someone who tends toward fluid accumulation, nettle could be helpful. If you are someone who is dry and has trouble hanging on to fluids, nettle could dry you out a little and therefore may not be the best choice for you. Watch for headaches and a dry mouth as a sign that it's too drying for you, and drink water to rectify (see Cautions).

NETTLE SAUERKRAUT   *Makes 2 quarts*

You'll need to gather about half a grocery bag full of nettles for this recipe. Wear gloves when harvesting and chopping the nettles, and if you are concerned about getting stung while preparing this recipe, you can beat the cabbage and nettles with a mallet, clean jar, or other tool. But I use my hands to massage the veggies and haven't had any problems. Be sure to thoroughly wash all equipment (jars, bowls, knives, cutting board, etc.) with hot water and soap before you begin. Using a food processor will greatly speed up the time it takes to finely chop the cabbage, onion, and carrots, but chop the nettles by hand and keep them separate.

This recipe was contributed by Diana Law, an herbalist and teacher in the Seattle area who is a passionate medicine maker, artist, and gardener. Find her online at dianaverse.org.

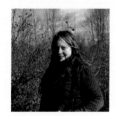

Diana Law

6 cups coarsely chopped fresh stinging nettle leaves
4 teaspoons kosher salt or sea salt
1 large green cabbage (about 3 pounds), very finely chopped
2 to 3 medium carrots, grated
1 small yellow onion, finely chopped
1 grape leaf or blackberry leaf, or 2 strawberry leaves (optional)

Put the nettles into a large bowl with 2 teaspoons of the salt. Add the cabbage, carrots, and onion to the bowl with the another 2 teaspoons salt.

Massage the veggies with your hands for 5 to 10 minutes, until they begin to release their juices.

Stuff the mixture into two quart-size jars and press firmly until the juices flow over the top of the cabbage. Top with a grape leaf to keep it crunchy. Be sure the

Because of its high mineral content, nettle leaf is recommended for hair, tooth, and bone health. It's a great source of calcium and iron in particular, but it also contains good amounts of boron, phosphorus, manganese, zinc, copper, magnesium, and others. Nettle is also found in many formulations for iron deficiency and menstruation. For this, it is often combined with other mineral-rich plants like alfalfa and horsetail.

Many cultures have used nettle stings as a remedy for joint pain, especially for the knees. To do this, take a bouquet of the spring leaves and whip the area of the body that you are treating. I don't recommend doing this with more sensitive areas like the neck or pelvic area. Knees, elbows, ankles, and wrists are excellent candidates. The stings will trigger an inflammatory response, which can help increase circulation and promote

liquid completely covers the kraut. I typically add a smaller jar filled with water as a weight, or a glass fermentation weight, which helps keep the cabbage below the brine level.

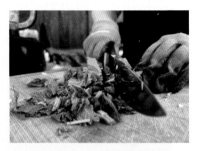

Cover the jar with cloth and a rubber band or air lock. It's important that the bacteria is able to breathe or the mixture will become anaerobic and rot. Some people use closed containers and "burp" their jars every day, but it's easy to forget about it and end up having to toss it, which is a shame with those lovely foraged nettles.

Set the jar aside on a dish to catch any overflow for 1 week, minimum. Check on it periodically, pressing down the weight to keep the cabbage below the brine surface. It should be kept out of the sunlight at a consistent temperature. Letting it sit longer makes a more "sauer" kraut. Once the kraut is sour enough for your taste, remove and discard the top leaves, and pick off any signs of mold. This is a wild, fermented food, and thus care must be taken not to cultivate the wrong bacteria in your ferment. If you feel like the taste or smell is off, throw it out.

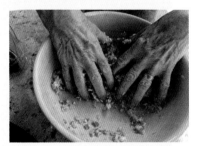

To store the kraut, seal the jars with lids and store in the refrigerator. The kraut will keep for 3 to 4 weeks. You will know it has gone bad when it starts producing an unappetizing, ammonia-like smell or if there is visible mold.

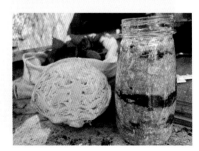

healing. I have tried this on my wrists and knees, and it definitely is quite the experience!

The medicinal use of nettle seed is fairly specific. Nettle seeds have an affinity for the kidneys and everything that goes along with kidney health. Nettle seeds are used to boost male and female fertility (fertility is associated with the kidneys in Chinese medicine) and to promote youthfulness (good kidney health equals strong qi). Like nettle leaves, the seeds are used to promote hair growth and can be taken for alopecia and other types of hair loss.

I like to share this urban legend when talking about nettle seed: It is said that Irish horse breeders used to feed nettle seed to their older horses before selling them. The nettle seed would make their hair shiny and give the old guys a pep in their step that made them seem much younger than they actually were. A little underhanded, but actually quite good for the horses!

Nettle seeds are also used for prostate inflammation. I have given nettle seed with celery seed tincture for gout (a kidney disorder) with a lot of success, and some herbalists have used nettle seed for chronic kidney failure. The seeds are also used for hypothyroid issues.

Nettle seed is less drying than the leaf and much more moistening. In fact, a tincture made from fresh nettle seed produces a large gelatinous mass. I recommend drying the seeds before working with them. They contain quite a few fatty acids, akin to chia and hemp seeds. This also means that nettle seed preparations go rancid quickly, so use the tincture and the dried seeds within a year.

A teaspoonful of ground dried nettle seeds is the recommended dose. Some people suggest you sprinkle it on your cereal or oatmeal in the morning. I don't find that enjoyable, so I'd sooner put it in a capsule or just mix it with some honey and chomp it down. I also enjoy nettle seed tea immensely, though you will miss out on some of the nutrition by not consuming the actual seeds.

Nettle root is used mostly for genitourinary-tract inflammation, especially prostate inflammation. For this, it is most often used as a tea or in capsules.

Making Medicine with Nettle

All parts of the nettle plant can be tinctured: the leaf, the seed, and the root (see Tincture Ratio Chart).

To dry nettle leaves for tea or other projects, spread your nettles out on a drying rack so they are touching as little as possible. Nettles dry pretty easily as long as they are not wet to start with.

When working with fresh nettles, you can keep them in a bag in the fridge for a few days before you use them. When using them for food, I blanch them for one minute in boiling water, grab them out with tongs, and squeeze them out under cold water. They will not sting you at this point, as the boiling water will have disarmed any stings. You can then freeze them or chop them up for a stir-fry or a soup. If you are not going to blanch them, make sure to chop them well and squish them up a bit to disarm the stings. I do this if I'm using fresh nettle in a stir-fry, for instance.

Cautions

Nettle seeds are known to be stimulating, so avoid taking them before bed, and don't take more than 1 ounce of seeds in a day. Nettle leaf can be quite drying, so limit use if you tend to be dry or dehydrated, and drink a lot of water when taking nettle. I have encountered nettle allergies in a few people, which seems to manifest as a mild-to-severe full-body rash (much like getting stung by nettles). Avoid nettles in all forms if you react to them.

Oregon Grape

Mahonia aquifolium, M. nervosa, M. repens
Berberidaceae (barberry family)

This plant is probably the most valuable medicine we have in our region, and we are lucky that it grows abundantly here. It is one of the best herbal antimicrobials I have used! We have three native species of *Mahonia* in our region and some ornamental species that do well in gardens.

Low Oregon grape (*Mahonia nervosa*) grows in forest understories mostly on the west side of the Cascades. East of the Cascades, it is much smaller and the leaves are redder. As the name suggests, low Oregon grape is much shorter than other species.

Tall Oregon grape (*Mahonia aquifolium*) prefers open areas with drier, rocky soils, like prairies and fields. It is found in both dry and wet parts of our bioregion. It is also a popular plant in drought-tolerant gardens as it requires very little water to survive. You can grab one at the nursery or propagate one with a cutting. Put your plant in a dry and sunny spot. Tall Oregon grape is also commonly used in public landscaping.

The third species is creeping Oregon grape (*Mahonia repens*), which grows exclusively east of the Cascades. Find it in forests dominated by ponderosa pine and lodgepole pine as well as sagebrush steppes. I have not used this species for medicine,

LEFT Low Oregon grape in flower **RIGHT** Tall Oregon grape

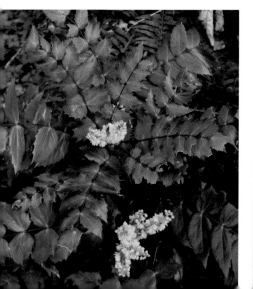
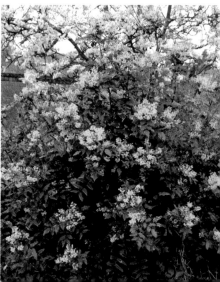

Tall Oregon grape
Mahonia aquifolium

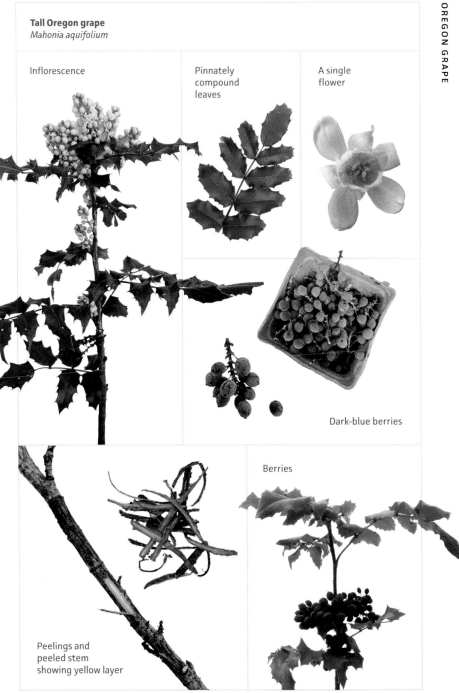

Inflorescence

Pinnately compound leaves

A single flower

Dark-blue berries

Berries

Peelings and peeled stem showing yellow layer

as it is usually quite small, and I have such good access to the other two.

Botanists recently decided that the plants in the genus *Mahonia* should go into the larger *Berberis* genus. This type of genus consolidation is part of a larger movement toward using gene sequencing to more accurately categorize plants. However, *Mahonia* are so morphologically distinct from *Berberis* that many have continued to use the *Mahonia* name. You may see these plants referred to as *Berberis aquifolium* and *Berberis nervosa* in some sources.

Harvesting Oregon Grape

I harvest the stem bark of tall Oregon grape because it does not require uprooting the plant. Once mature, a tall Oregon grape plant often has more than ten woody stalks. To harvest, select a branch thicker than your thumb and use clippers or a saw to cut it. It's best to cut right after a node, where a smaller branch forks off. That way, the energy that was going into the branch you remove will go into the smaller branch. On occasion, I have been fortunate enough to see park staff trimming tall Oregon grape hedges in city parks and have asked to take some branches home from the pile. A great source indeed!

Should you choose to harvest the root of tall Oregon grape, find the roots that run parallel to the surface of the ground by digging around the plant. Sever the root and get as much out of the ground as you can, leaving the main plant intact.

With low Oregon grape, because of its growth habit, we harvest the bark from the aboveground stems and belowground roots. This method of harvesting kills the plant, so I harvest only from very abundant patches, choosing the most crowded areas within a patch to harvest from. If there are only a few plants, please skip the harvest. To harvest, seize the base of the stem and pull gently to get as much root out of the ground as possible. Be careful not to fall backward when it breaks! The roots grow parallel to the ground under the soft leaf duff until they plunge into the soil. Several plants usually branch off from the same root stock.

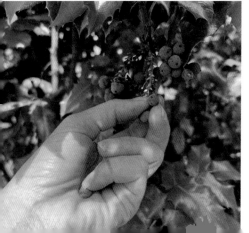

Harvesting tall Oregon grape berries to make jelly in early July at sea level

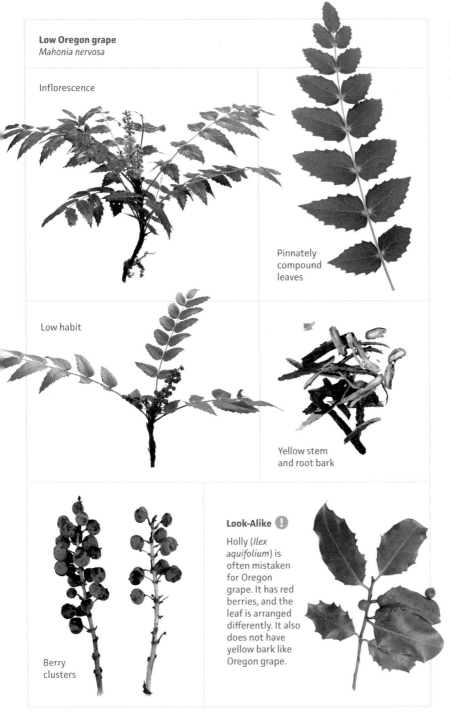

Low Oregon grape
Mahonia nervosa

Inflorescence

Pinnately compound leaves

Low habit

Yellow stem and root bark

Berry clusters

Look-Alike ❗

Holly (*Ilex aquifolium*) is often mistaken for Oregon grape. It has red berries, and the leaf is arranged differently. It also does not have yellow bark like Oregon grape.

When you get your sticks home, remove the lichen and moss by scraping with the back of a butter knife or a scrub brush. Use water only if you must. Once clean, peel the bark off with a pocketknife, holding the knife perpendicular to the stem and peeling away from yourself. Peel off only the outer, brown layer and the bright-yellow bark underneath it; stop peeling where it turns white. The white part is the wood, which is not medicinal.

The berries, which ripen around July, are edible and incredibly sour due to their high vitamin C content. A jelly made from Oregon grape berries, sweetened with sugar to enhance the flavor of the berries, is delicious (see Oregon Grape Jelly). I also like to eat the bitter flower buds as a trail snack.

Medicinal Uses of Oregon Grape

Most of the medicinal uses of Oregon grape revolve around its antimicrobial properties. An antimicrobial is something that kills or discourages bacteria, viruses, fungus, and any other microbes. I was once sitting with students in a silent meditation with Oregon grape. The forest was dark, and we were surrounded by a tangled canopy of cedar boughs and bigleaf maple. The plants themselves were hemmed in by a thick mat of rotting bigleaf maple leaves. It was at that moment that I fully appreciated the antimicrobial qualities of Oregon grape; the roots of the plant have to survive in a dark, rotting place all year long without rotting themselves. What a feat!

On top of being a great antimicrobial, Oregon grape is also a biofilm disruptor. Biofilms are like veils that bacterial and fungal colonies wear to protect themselves from immune responses and antimicrobial substances. The tenacity of many chronic bacterial and fungal infections can be attributed to biofilms.

This herb works best when there is direct contact with the infected site. That means that it is ideal for gut infections and skin infections. It can be used for urinary tract infections, especially if consumed with water. It is also a great remedy for food poisoning, so I always carry Oregon grape tincture when I travel. You can even take it preventatively if you think something you ate was funky, or as soon as you start to feel an upset stomach. My dose for this is 3 dropperfuls of Oregon grape tincture in 8 fluid ounces of water. I take that up to 8 times a day depending on the severity (see Cautions). Continue this high dose for only 1 to 3 days, and then follow through with 3 doses a day for another 3 days.

Oregon grape can be used for conjunctivitis: make a hot infusion of the stem bark, wait for it to cool, and dip a sterile wound dressing or cloth in it to make a compress. No need to keep the eye open for this, just hold it on the closed eye for a minute or two, then soak the cloth again and repeat a few times. A few applications should be enough, but for more persistent cases, 3 to 5 applications a day for a few days should do it. You can also use this preparation for styes.

You can use Oregon grape tincture on cuts to prevent them from getting infected. You could even add it to a 1-ounce spray bottle and spray it on.

For even more antimicrobial power, mix Oregon grape with different berberine-containing plants in a formula. This is based on the principle that the more diverse the set of compounds fighting an infection, the more difficult it is for the microbes to adapt and fight back.

FRESH OREGON GRAPE BARK TINCTURE   *Makes 4 to 5 ounces*

Using fresh bark for this recipe makes for a more potent tincture. Not only that, but store-bought Oregon grape bark often includes the wood and is therefore less concentrated. Scrape the bark off the stems or roots. I scrape with a butter knife held at a 90-degree angle to the stem. The bark ends up in much smaller pieces, which make for a better extraction. If you have more than you need for the recipe, you can scale up the amount of alcohol accordingly. This recipe dilutes 95 percent alcohol with water to create a 60 percent alcohol solution.

Dosage: Take 30 to 60 drops 1 to 10 times a day, depending on application.

1.25 ounces fresh Oregon grape stem bark
3 fluid ounces 190-proof alcohol
  (95 percent), such as Everclear
2 fluid ounces water

Put the bark in a clean 8-ounce jar. Pour the alcohol and water over the bark.
  Seal the jar with the lid and label well.
  Let sit in a cool, dark place for 4 weeks. Shake a few times while macerating. Strain it through cheesecloth and store in an 8-ounce jar in a cool, dark place for up to 5 years.

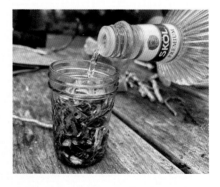

THE PLANTS AND RECIPES

OREGON GRAPE JELLY *Makes 6 cups*

This is a standard jelly recipe using liquid pectin. I have made it three years in a row and the recipe has held up consistently. This recipe was given to me by Elise Krohn (wildfoodsandmedicines.com), an herbalist, native foods specialist, educator, and author with more than twenty years of experience. She currently works and teaches at GRuB (Garden-Raised Bounty) in Olympia, Washington. Make sure to harvest the berries when they are deep blue. They will still be tart, but less so than unripe berries.

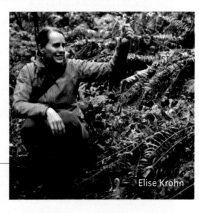

Elise Krohn

6 cups Oregon grape berries,
  cleaned and rinsed
2 cups water, plus more as needed
1 ounce pectin (about half of
  a liquid package)
2 tablespoons freshly squeezed lemon juice
3 cups granulated cane sugar

Place the berries in a large pot with the water.
  Bring to a boil, then turn down and simmer for 15 minutes. Use a large spoon to mash the berries against the side of the pot so the juice is released.
  Place a food mill over another cooking pot. In 1-to-2-cup increments, turn the berries and juice through the food mill so that the seeds are separated. Remove the seeds from the mill before straining another batch.
  Once finished, you should have approximately 3 cups of juice/pulp. If you have less,

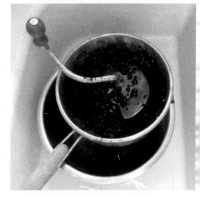

Photo by Elise Krohn

you can add a little water to bring your volume to 3 cups.
  Place a pot on the stovetop. Add the berry juice and pulp, pectin, and lemon juice. Stir well and then cook over high heat, stirring constantly.
  Once the mixture is boiling, rapidly stir in the sugar, return to a rolling boil, and boil for exactly 1 minute. Remove from the burner.
  Transfer the jelly to jars and store in the fridge for immediate use. Use within 3 weeks. Or pour the jelly into plastic freezer jars and freeze. The jelly will keep in the freezer for up to 6 months.

There has been a lot of research done on Oregon grape as a topical treatment for psoriasis and atopic dermatitis with fairly promising results. It is also used internally for both eczema and psoriasis with other classic herbs like yellow dock root and burdock root.

Making Medicine with Oregon Grape

The most typical and useful preparation of Oregon grape is a tincture of the stem bark (see Fresh Oregon Grape Bark Tincture). Berberine is very soluble in alcohol, and a tincture preserves the medicine very well. The tincture can be used internally and externally. For external use, to temper the effect of the alcohol, you can wet a cotton round and put 5 to 10 drops of Oregon grape tincture on it.

Berberine breaks down when heated, so be sure to steep it in hot water rather than boiling it on the stove, as you normally would for a bark or root. I make a hot infusion of Oregon grape for compresses and wound soaks.

I find people are often tempted to make an Oregon grape salve, which I do not recommend. Berberine and other constituents are alcohol soluble, not oil soluble, and therefore not effective in that format. Pine resin salve is a much better option if you are looking for an antimicrobial salve.

Though you could purchase dried Oregon grape bark to use to make medicine, the dried bark from commercial sources will include the inner wood along with the bark. You can tell because there will be yellow and white pieces. When you harvest it yourself, you have the ability to peel off just the bark, yielding a far stronger product.

Cautions

Oregon grape is an herb to take on a short-term basis, I would say 6 weeks at a time. I typically don't exceed more than 3 dropperfuls of tincture in one dose, and would take that dose up to 8 times a day only for very acute cases. Watch for headaches or abdominal sensations, which are subtle indications that your body has had a bit too much.

Pine

Pinus ponderosa, P. contorta, P. monticola
Pinaceae (pine family)

People often call all evergreens "pine" trees. Botanically speaking, the name should be reserved for members of the *Pinus* genus, which is part of the pine family. All members of this genus have needles that are grouped together with a membrane, creating a packet of needles called a fascicle. Depending on the species, each fascicle will contain one to seven needles. We have three common pine trees in Washington: white pine (*Pinus monticola*) has five needles, ponderosa pine (*Pinus ponderosa*) has three, and lodgepole pine (*Pinus contorta*) has two. All three of these pines grow primarily in the western US.

White pines are actually a group of several different species, our native western white pine being just one of them. They all have elongated pine cones and packets of five needles. It is common to find other species of white pine planted in parks and yards—these are actually the species I end up harvesting.

Lodgepole pines have two twisted needles per fascicle, hence the name *contorta*. The common name, lodgepole, comes from the trunks of these trees, which are straight as a pin. Lodgepole pines are dependent on fire in that their seeds require fire to germinate. Ironically, the trees themselves are not that fire resistant, having quite thin bark. They are also a target of pine beetles, which kill whole stands of trees and set the stage for high-intensity fires. There are several subspecies of lodgepole pine, two of which are distinct and common in our region: The first is shore pine (*Pinus contorta* subsp. *contorta*), which you can see decorating the bluffs of the Pacific coast, the trunks and branches gnarled and bent by wind and erosion. The second is lodgepole pine (*Pinus contorta* subsp. *latifolia*), which prefers dry mountain forests.

Ponderosa pine forests are common east of the Cascades and were

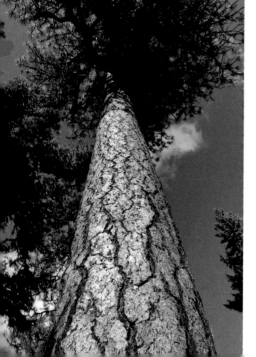

An old ponderosa pine with thick bark and high limbs to help it survive fire

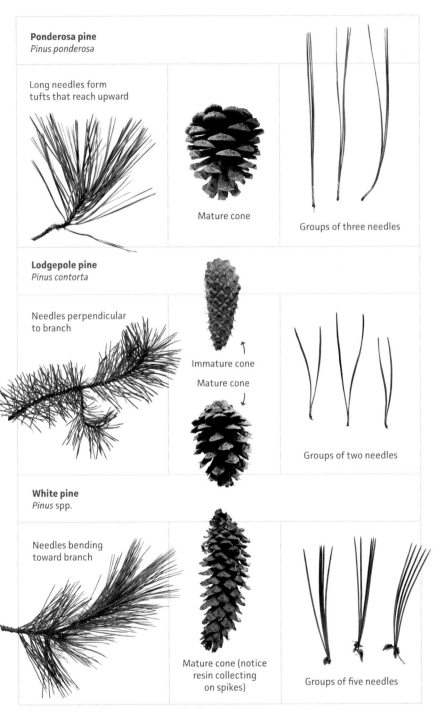

Ponderosa pine
Pinus ponderosa

Long needles form
tufts that reach upward

Mature cone

Groups of three needles

Lodgepole pine
Pinus contorta

Needles perpendicular
to branch

Immature cone

Mature cone

Groups of two needles

White pine
Pinus spp.

Needles bending
toward branch

Mature cone (notice
resin collecting
on spikes)

Groups of five needles

traditionally managed with prescribed burning by local Native groups. Prescribed burning is a practice in which people intentionally start low-intensity forest fires to burn away the grass and underbrush. These burns increase the production of several significant food crops, including camas, huckleberries, and bracken fern root. Ponderosa pines have a number of amazing adaptations to fire, allowing them to survive these low-intensity prescribed burns.

Colonization and subsequent shifts from Indigenous land-management practices to modern agriculture and private land ownership have significantly changed the fire ecology of ponderosa pine forests and other types of forests. When fires are infrequent, dead underbrush, shrubs, and young trees (known as "ladder fuels") accumulate. When fire does come along, the flames climb the ladder fuels and get high enough to reach the canopy of older trees and can kill entire forests. The high temperatures these fires reach also kill seeds, fungal associates, perennial roots, insects, and small animals that the forest relies on to regenerate itself after a fire.

Prescribed burning is already being reintroduced as a forest management technique, both by the forest service and local tribes. I hope to see more of it in the future!

LEFT A few good chunks of ponderosa pine resin found in icy November **RIGHT** Harvesting ponderosa pine pollen

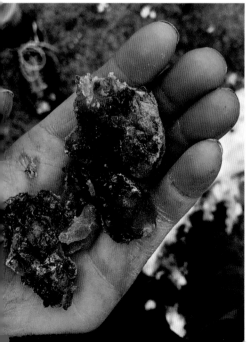 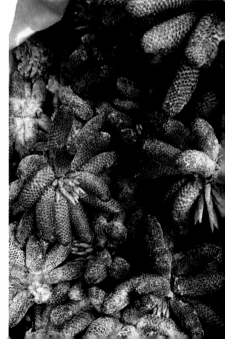

Harvesting Pine

You can harvest the needles of all species of pine for tea. The younger ones are tastiest. They emerge at the ends of the branches in spring and are best harvested in May or June. White pine needles are the best tasting of our local pines and make a delicious tea fresh or dried. Ponderosa pine and lodgepole pine both have a more turpentine flavor, so avoid using those for tea.

Pine pollen is ready around April or May, depending on the elevation. Ponderosa pine has the easiest pollen to harvest because its pollen structures are large and grouped. Lodgepole pine pollen is also fairly easy to harvest, though its pollen structures are smaller and slightly more dispersed. Pick them off like fruit just as they're opening and put them all in a bag, which will catch the pollen as it is released. Sift the particulate out of the pollen using a fine-mesh strainer. Store pine pollen in the freezer as it does not keep well.

Lodgepole pine tends to have epically large globs of resin that make it the easiest pine to harvest resin from. These globs can be harvested at any time of year. Avoid exposing any wounds on the tree that the glob may have been covering. I frequently harvest from ponderosa pines as well because I like their resin in particular.

The bark of white pine is the only pine-family bark that I harvest. The bark from the others can be flaky and too strong in flavor, whereas white pine bark is aromatic, sweet, and easy to peel from the branches. I harvest it from branches the diameter of a broom handle. Harvest in April or May and it should peel off in huge, wet pieces. The peeled bark smells like tropical fruit.

I also harvest fallen ponderosa pine needles to make coil baskets, which are time-consuming but incredibly beautiful. Find a tree with the longest needles possible (certain trees have longer needles than others). From the ground, select recently fallen needles that have a red or tan color and are unbroken.

Medicinal Uses of Pine

Pine, even more than spruce or fir, is highly antimicrobial. It is a superlative first aid plant because you can almost always find it nearby when you're out in the field, and it can be used for all kinds of infections. A wound soak using a decoction of pine needles or bark would be great for an infection, even for an animal bite or scratch. Pine has been used historically for urinary tract infections, though that use has fallen out of favor in modern times. Pine preparations can also be used to control *H. pylori* infections in the stomach.

PINE RESIN SALVE
Makes eight 0.5-ounce jars or tins

This salve is one of the salves I use most often. I use it to discourage infection in cuts and scrapes, but also to help resolve pimples more quickly. If you are feeling extra crafty, you could even put it into lip balm tubes (for which you will need a higher ratio of beeswax), making it easier to apply.

Dosage: Rub onto cuts or healing wounds a few times a day.

3.5 fluid ounces organic extra-virgin olive oil
0.5 ounce pine resin
0.5 ounce beeswax pastilles

Set up a double boiler (a.k.a. bain-marie): in a medium saucepan, add 1 to 2 inches of water.

Grab a clean, old 8-ounce jar (one that you don't mind discarding at the end of the project), and pour the oil into the jar. Put the pan on the stove, place the jar in the pan, and adjust the level of water to match the level of oil in the jar. Turn the heat to medium. Add the resin to the oil.

As the water gets hot, use a chopstick to stir for about 5 minutes. Adjust the heat as needed to maintain a gentle bubble. During this time, the resin will start to get sticky and dissolve, and eventually a solid brown mass will form. Remove this with the chopstick and set aside on a paper towel or piece of newspaper. This can be used later as a fire starter!

Add the beeswax to the jar and stir until totally dissolved. Remove from the heat and pour immediately as it will start hardening in the jar.

Pour the mixture into eight 0.5-ounce jars and let sit uncovered until they harden. Cover and store in a cool, dry place for up to 3 years.

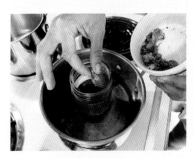 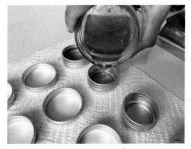

Hot pine-needle tea can help dislodge and expel phlegm and kill a secondary bacterial infection in the lungs. You can also use pine in sinus steams for sinus infections or just stuck phlegm. If you are prone to sinus infections, try an occasional pine-needle steam while you have a cold or during allergy season, as preventing is much easier than treating an active infection.

Pine pollen has been described by some as "herbal vitamins." It contains B vitamins, proteins, and several minerals. I like to snack on it a bit on the trail during pollen season. It has also recently become popular as a "male tonic," supposedly helping raise low testosterone levels. Pine pollen is considered a phytotestosterone, which is a plant that mimics testosterone in the body, though whether it actually works to boost testosterone levels is rather controversial. The testosterone industry is lucrative and certainly benefits from overhyping the effects of supplements. That said, a lot of people swear by it, including some herbalists, so there might be something to it.

Pine resin salve is a great remedy to have in your apothecary. It is highly antimicrobial and very effective for preventing and treating minor infections in wounds. It is also used for arthritic pain. It is warming and a little irritating, which increases blood circulation. In herbalism, we see arthritis not as one disease but as having many different possible qualities. Pine resin could be a great remedy for "cold" joints, which are worse with cold weather and tend to have a fixed, dull ache. For "hot" joints, the pain may be exacerbated because pine is warming.

Turpentine—a refined product from pine resin—is extracted in large quantities using a certain chevron-like cut in the trunk of the tree. A vessel is placed at the base of the cut to collect the dripping resin. In addition to being a solvent for painters and boat makers, turpentine was once widely used as medicine. All kinds of wild claims were made about its benefits, and it was even sold by traveling circus shows. Now it is known to be dangerous to ingest, causing kidney damage and bleeding in the lungs. This, along with other dangerous herbal remedies of that era, is one of the reasons that product claims are now heavily regulated.

Making Medicine with Pine

Pine needles can be made into a hot infusion or a decoction. I have also made white-pine-needle elixir (soak needles in a menstruum of honey and alcohol). Pine needles also make a great sinus steam. To do this, put a few handfuls of needles in a pot of hot water and lean over it with a towel over your head, then inhale the steam for a couple of minutes.

You can also make a hydrosol out of pine needles, and with the right equipment, you can capture the essential oil. I typically buy the essential oil and use it in homemade cleaning supplies.

Pine resin can be applied directly to the skin. It can also be dissolved in oil and made into salves or creams (see Pine Resin Salve).

Pine bark can be boiled in water and applied as a wash.

Pine pollen can be made into a tincture, put into capsules, or added to smoothies or baked goods.

Cautions

Resin from pine-family trees, including spruce, should not be taken internally in doses exceeding 30 drops of standardized tincture in one day, as it can result in kidney damage or joint pain. Use caution even when taking small amounts, such as 10 drops of the tincture. Historical accounts refer to pine resin being used internally, but that does not necessarily mean it is safe.

Do not consume any part of pine when pregnant. Do not take pine bark internally for long periods or in large doses.

Plantain

Plantago major, P. lanceolata
Plantaginaceae (plantain family)

There are two main species of plantain in our region: broadleaf plantain (*Plantago major*) and narrowleaf plantain (*Plantago lanceolata*). These have nothing to do with the starchy, banana-like fruit.

Both broadleaf and narrowleaf plantain were brought to North America from Europe by colonists and quickly naturalized and spread across the continent. Some states consider one or both species to be a noxious weed, though usually a low priority. In the Pacific Northwest, we do have a few native species of the same genus, but they are not as common and don't necessarily have the same uses.

Broadleaf plantain loves to grow along hiking trails and in gravel paths, driveways, and lawns—it seems to thrive on being driven over and stepped on. It's a bit of an herbalist's joke, in fact. Narrowleaf plantain is more commonly found in grassy meadows and open weedy areas. Broadleaf plantain is found both east and west of the Cascades, whereas narrowleaf is found more on the west side of the mountains, where it's a bit wetter.

LEFT Narrowleaf plantain coming up near a parking lot **RIGHT** Broadleaf plantain growing in one of its favorite habitats: lawn

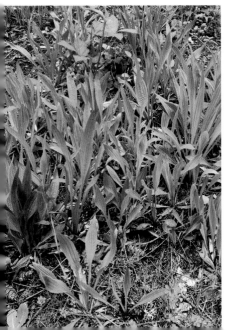 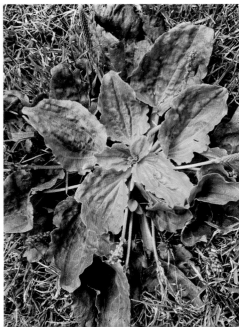

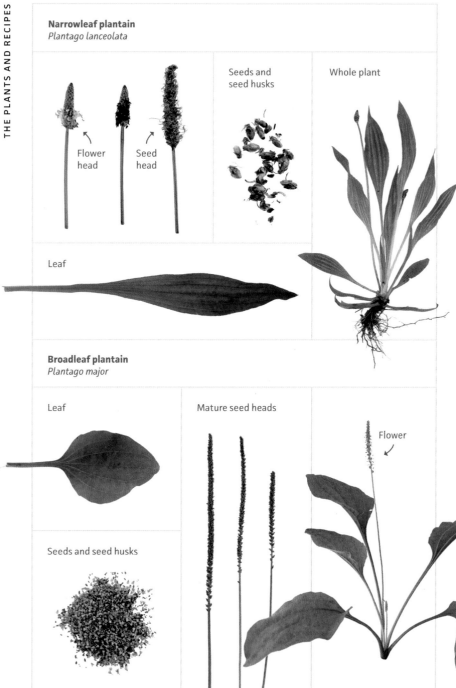

Narrowleaf plantain
Plantago lanceolata

Flower
head

Seed
head

Seeds and
seed husks

Whole plant

Leaf

Broadleaf plantain
Plantago major

Leaf

Mature seed heads

Flower

Seeds and seed husks

Harvesting Plantain

Always harvest plantain on a dry day. To harvest the leaves of plantain, I crop each leaf off at the base with my thumbnail. Sometimes you can get scissors and snip multiple leaves at once, or snip off whole plants. Plantain is an abundant and non-native weed in our area, so this practice is okay for this particular plant, much like dandelion.

If you plan to dry the plantain leaves, it is imperative that you harvest on the driest possible day. Using a food dehydrator is best, but even a fan trained on your drying rack for the first twenty-four hours would speed up the process. If the leaves dry too slowly, or if they're damp, black gooey polymers form on the surface of the leaves. The polymers are not toxic, but the resulting leaves are soft and look moldy. Commercial plantain leaf is dried in large driers to prevent this.

Harvesting a particularly large broad-leaf plantain leaf

For harvesting seeds and husks, I prefer broadleaf plantain as there are more per plant and the harvest is easier. They are ripe in late August and all through September. Wait until the seed stalks are brown (but not black with mold), and choose a nice dry day for your harvest. Grip the stalk at the base, where the seeds begin, and pull upward, stripping the seeds into your hand. There will be light seed husks and tiny seeds. Use all of it. You can also clip the seed stalks off, put them in a bag, and strip them at home. Also note that there are often tiny insects hiding among the seeds in the stalk, so give the little guys a chance to crawl out. For drying the seeds, I typically fold a piece of paper to make a small tray to keep them in as they can easily blow away.

Medicinal Uses of Plantain

Both narrowleaf and broadleaf plantain have generally the same uses, so I refer to both here as *plantain*. Plantain leaf is soothing, anti-inflammatory, and vulnerary (a medicine that speeds wound healing).

The handiest use of plantain leaf is as a spit poultice for insect bites, rashes, and nettle stings. A spit poultice is made by chewing the fresh leaf carefully, then spitting the green pulp onto the affected area. You can put a leaf on top of the poultice and tie a piece of grass over it to keep it in place. You can also use an infused oil topically for the same afflictions. It is an absolute game changer for rashes of any kind, and I highly recommend

PLANTAIN AND CALENDULA FIRST AID SALVE *Makes four 1-ounce tins*

This salve is excellent for burns, rashes, bug bites, and wounds. It is soothing, vulnerary (heals wounds), and slightly antimicrobial. I commonly use it on nettle stings. Store a small tin in your herbal first aid kit so you have it when needed. For this recipe, you can use infused oils made the traditional way or using the alcohol-intermediary-oil method. You can also purchase the infused oils if you need to. I use beeswax pastilles because they are uniform in size and melt quickly, but you can use grated beeswax if that's what you have.

Dosage: Apply to cuts, scrapes, or rashes 2 to 3 times a day.

3.5 fluid ounces calendula infused oil
3.5 fluid ounces plantain leaf infused oil
1 ounce beeswax pastilles

Lay out a paper towel or newspaper on the counter and arrange your salve tins on top of it, lids off, so that they are ready to be filled.

Put the oils and beeswax into an old, clean 16-ounce jar. The jar is very hard to clean, so I often end up tossing it out after using it.

Add a couple of inches of water to a medium saucepan. Place the jar in the saucepan and adjust the water level to ensure that it matches the level of oil in the jar.

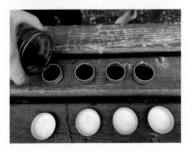

Put the pan on a burner on the stovetop over medium heat. As the water heats up, use a chopstick to stir the mixture until all the beeswax has melted. This should take 5 to 10 minutes.

Once melted, carefully pour the salve into each tin. Let sit, uncovered, until the salve has hardened. Then put the lids on and label. Keep the tins in a cool, dark location for up to 2 years.

adding a plantain salve to your first aid kit. For a first aid salve for burns and wounds, calendula flower and plantain leaf are a classic combo.

Plantain also helps draw pus out of wounds and can be used for wound healing and infection as a fresh leaf poultice. I have a friend who used a fresh leaf poultice with success on her small dog who had gotten bitten by another dog. Of course, you need to make sure the infection is being addressed in other ways too, if it's a serious one.

Plantain is effective for internal wounds and inflammation as well. Gastrointestinal (GI) tract issues that involve wounding or eroding the GI lining are a great place for plantain to do its work. If you have a food sensitivity and have had an exposure, a blend with plantain can help your inflamed gut recover more quickly. For an irritated and inflamed GI tract, I make a tea of plantain leaf, chamomile flower, marshmallow root, and calendula flower. You can even put it in a tea formula for reflux.

Plantain is also often used in cough formulas to soothe dry coughs and as an expectorant for stuck coughs. Mullein is a great pairing for this use. For a dry cough, I make a tea of plantain leaf, marshmallow root, licorice root, and wild cherry bark. For an irritated cough with stubborn, dry phlegm, I make a tea of mullein, plantain leaf, elderflower, and thyme.

Psyllium husk, a popular bulk-forming laxative, comes from a species of plantain that grows in India. The husks of broadleaf and narrowleaf plantain can be used just like psyllium. They absorb water much like chia seeds, forming a gel-like matrix of long-chain polysaccharides. Dry the husks first, and then either grind them or keep them whole. I recommend grinding them; they are easier to swallow as a powder. Combine 1 teaspoon of ground husks with 8 fluid ounces of water, stir, and drink immediately. Do this once a day before bed to regulate bowel movement and soften stool. If you don't take plantain husk with enough water, it may absorb water in your intestines and cause constipation.

Making Medicine with Plantain

I typically make hot infusions (tea) from the dried leaves, usually with other herbs (see Medicinal Uses of Plantain for some suggestions). This can be consumed for internal uses, or cooled and used as a wash or compress on the skin.

STOMACH-SOOTHING TEA FORMULA *Makes about 1.5 ounces loose-leaf tea*

This is one of my favorite tea blends. It can be used for inflammation from food sensitivities as well as reflux and other burning conditions.

Dosage: Use 1 tablespoon per cup. Infuse for 10 minutes, covered. Drink 1 to 2 cups a day.

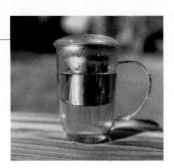

0.4 ounce dried marshmallow root
0.3 ounce dried plantain leaf
0.3 ounce dried chamomile flowers
0.25 ounce dried lemon balm
0.2 ounce dried licorice root

Combine all ingredients in a bowl. Mix well. Store in a 12-ounce jar for up to 2 years.

You can make a lovely green alcohol intermediary oil from the dried leaves (see Bleeding Heart Alcohol Intermediary Oil for directions). I use olive oil for this, but almond oil would be a nice combination as well. From there, you can make a salve and even add other oils to it for a formula. A classic combination is plantain leaf oil and calendula flower oil (see Plantain and Calendula First Aid Salve).

You can also make a traditional infused oil from fresh plantain leaf using the hot-water-bath method (see Cottonwood Bud Infused Oil). You will need to wilt the leaves first for about twenty-four hours. To wilt leaves, leave them out on a towel or basket and allow them to become floppy.

To prepare plantain seeds to use for their prebiotic and bulking fiber properties, add 1 teaspoon of ground plantain seeds (with husks) to 4 to 8 ounces of water, stir briefly, and drink quickly before it has a chance to get too solid. Do this every day before bed. Avoid taking the seeds and husks without water, as they soak up water and can cause constipation.

Red Clover

Trifolium pratense
Fabaceae (pea family)

Red clover is a non-native plant from Europe that has success-fully naturalized all over the country, including here in the Pacific Northwest. It is not an aggressive weed, but still quite common. Like other pea-family plants, it fixes nitrogen and can be used as a cover crop with the added benefit of having medicinal flowers for harvesting.

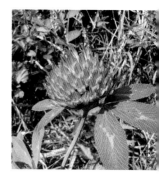

A blooming red clover

Most often, I find red clover growing in gardens where the soil has been disturbed and there is a little extra water. Like plantain, it seems to like to grow along edges, paths, and roads, but also in meadow-like grassy fields.

White clover is not used in herbal medicine much, though bees prefer it over red clover because of its more continuous bloom cycle. Leave it in your lawn for them!

Harvesting Red Clover

For medicine, harvest the flowers of red clover, which bloom from June through August. Snip off the freshest, brightest-pink flowers along with one set of leaves. I often end up harvesting these in small batches. Perhaps a handful in the park on a walk, another handful in a friend's garden, and another handful at a trailhead. I bring each handful home and put it in the des-ignated red clover area on my drying rack; it eventually adds up to quite a lot. Like calendula, red clover plants continue to flower and will flower more when harvested.

LEFT Gather red clover in batches as the flowers bloom and dry for tea in a basket or a drying rack. **RIGHT** Use scissors to harvest the flower and the top set of leaves.

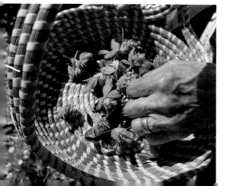
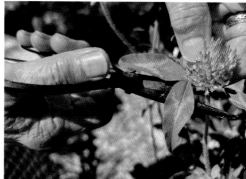

Single, tube-shaped floret

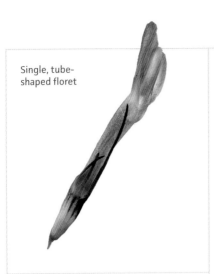

A compound inflorescence, made up of many tiny flowers

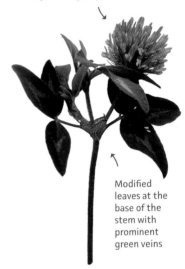

Modified leaves at the base of the stem with prominent green veins

Once pollinated, the flowers turn brown.

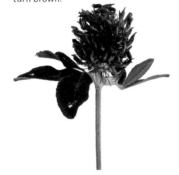

Look-Alike

White clover (*Trifolium repens*) has very similar leaves but is much shorter. It often grows in lawns.

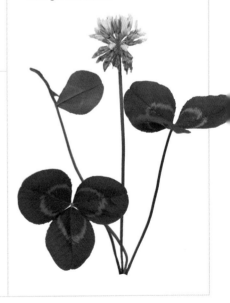

Three-lobed leaves, each with a light-green chevron

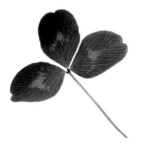

Medicinal Uses of Red Clover

Red clover has gained the most attention as a phytoestrogen. It has been found to contain many types of isoflavones, a type of secondary compound that resembles estradiol (a form of estrogen), and can bind to estrogen-receptor sites. Red clover can help lower estrogen levels by occupying receptor sites and blocking xenoestrogens from binding there. It can be used to increase low endogenous estrogen, as is often the case in menopause. Red clover is a great plant to try for menopausal hot flashes, a use which is supported by history and modern research.

The discovery of red clover's phytoestrogens seems to have pigeonholed the use of this plant to hormonal issues, but its uses are much more extensive. Red clover is a moistening, nutritive, and gently cleansing herb, acting primarily on the lymphatic system and lungs. It is considered an alterative, which is an herb that helps open channels of elimination in some way (bowel movements, urine, sweat, etc.). It is also an effective treatment for red, dry skin conditions such as eczema and psoriasis. For eczema, red clover is much gentler than yellow dock and is better suited for dry constitutions.

This plant was once used topically in various preparations on cancerous growths, especially breast cancer. One such preparation involved cooking down a paste of the flowers and applying the paste to the tumor, apparently to draw it out of the skin. I don't recommend this old, unpleasant remedy. Cancer is a serious disease, and herbs should not be relied upon as a sole treatment. Herbs are much better used as a preventative to promote good health and balance.

Making Medicine with Red Clover

I use dried red clover flowers in hot infusions, usually mixed with other herbs. For lymphatic congestion, combine red clover with cleavers and calendula in a tea. This is a very gentle formula, designed to work over time. Red clover can also be used for spasmodic coughs as a strong infusion. For this, combine it with herbs like wild cherry bark and thyme. It is also a great addition in tea for mild wildfire smoke exposure, which is fast becoming a seasonal occurrence in the Pacific Northwest. See the Wildfire Season Tea recipe for my favorite combination.

For eczema and other skin conditions with redness, dryness, and congestion, combine it in a tea with violet leaf and burdock.

You can make a tincture (see Tincture Ratio Chart), though I question the effectiveness of a gentle herb like this used in a tincture.

Cautions

Many sources caution against taking red clover while pregnant or breastfeeding because of its hormonal effects.

WILDFIRE SEASON TEA

Makes 1.2 ounces loose-leaf tea

I drink this tea to support my lungs during fire season, when the smoke is thick in the air. It is demulcent (soothing), gently expectorant, anti-inflammatory to lung tissue, and gently cleansing to the lymphatic system. It would also make a great daily tea for a smoker or for someone with a residual cough after illness. This also makes a delightful iced tea with honey. Strain this tea well before drinking so the mullein hairs don't irritate your throat.

As you measure each herb, garble the herbs, breaking them down to smaller pieces. To break up the mullein leaves, crush and rub them between your hands (see photo). The more energy you put into breaking them down, the more uniform your tea blend will be.

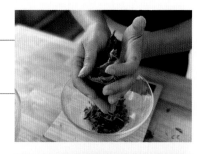

Dosage: Use 2 tablespoons per cup of boiling water. Infuse for 10 minutes, covered. Drink a cup or two every day when the smoke is bad.

0.5 ounce dried marshmallow root
0.3 ounce dried goldenrod flowers
0.2 ounce dried plantain leaf
0.1 ounce dried red clover flowers
0.1 ounce dried mullein leaf

In a large bowl, mix and massage all the herbs together with your hands.

Transfer to a 32-ounce jar and store in a cool, dark place for up to 2 years.

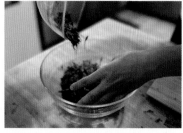

Red Root

Ceanothus velutinus
Rhamnaceae (buckthorn family)

This plant is better known as snowbrush ceanothus (*Ceanothus velutinus*). "Red root" is a common name favored by herbalists. There are more than sixty species of *Ceanothus* in the US, many of which are native to the Pacific Northwest. Species in the *Ceanothus* genus have a long history of medicinal use by Native groups all over North America.

Red root is an essential part of wildfire ecology in some of the more arid areas of the Pacific Northwest. This shrub's nitrogen-fixing root nodules increase the nitrogen content of the soil, which is lost during fires and needed for new trees to grow. Red root populations are strongest in the first ten years post-burn and are even able to survive catastrophic fires. The seeds survive in the soil for a few hundred years and need heat to germinate.

Red root's role in the ecosystem is actually quite similar to red alder: soil stabilization and nitrogen fixation. Interestingly, red alder also has red bark and similar medicinal uses.

Snowbrush ceanothus in full bloom east of the Cascades in Washington. These shrubs thrive in drier forests with frequent fire regimes.

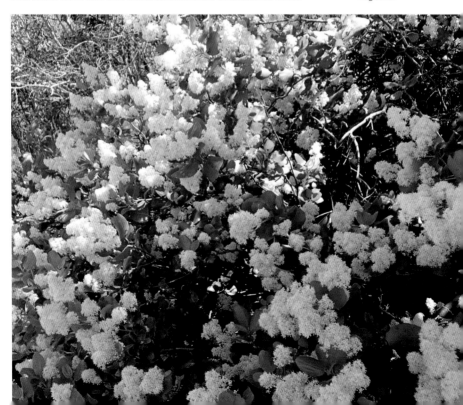

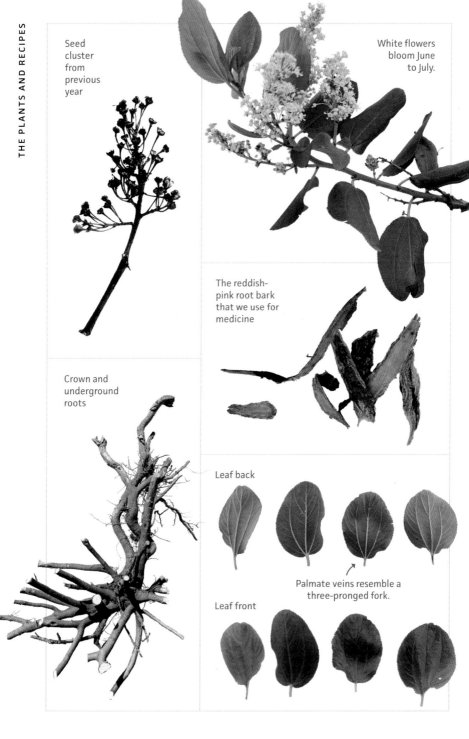

Seed cluster from previous year

White flowers bloom June to July.

The reddish-pink root bark that we use for medicine

Crown and underground roots

Leaf back

Palmate veins resemble a three-pronged fork.

Leaf front

Harvesting Red Root

There are four parts of the plant that you can harvest: the root bark, the stem bark, the leaves, and the flowers. A single red root bush is typically around 3 feet tall and between 4 and 7 feet in diameter. Branches can be up to 2 inches in diameter.

The root bark of red root is the classic part of this plant to harvest and use medicinally. The roots are best harvested after flowering, from August to January. I typically go out in September or October as my patches tend to get snow in the winter.

To unearth a root, you will need some type of pickax or mattock, gloves, and heavy-duty loppers used for tree pruning. Select a bush that stands alone without too many trees or other shrubs around it, and preferably in soil that isn't rock-solid. Choosing the right bush will make the job much easier. Begin

Digging for Red Root

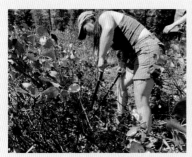

Cut the branches off the crown.

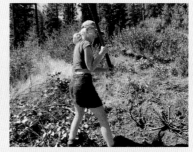

Dig around the crown to expose the root.

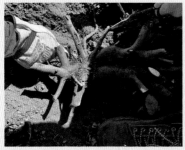

Use hands and small shovels to unearth specific roots.

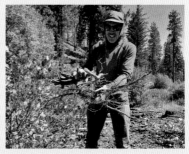

Saw off any stubborn roots, and voila!

by sawing or clipping off all the branches down to the ground, much like giving the bush a buzz cut. Keep the branches and leaves for medicine if you wish. Next, dig a ditch around the crown of the plant and start to dig down and around to find the root. I use a pickax for the initial digging process as shovels often have trouble penetrating the hard soils that red root prefers. Having several people working together makes the digging process go much faster. Then it's as simple as digging down and following the root as far as you can. At some point you'll get tired of digging, which is when you saw the root off and take what you have.

TINCTURE OF FRESH RED ROOT BARK *Makes 8 to 10 ounces*

Red root tincture should be made with fresh root bark for the most potent product. Peel the bark of the root off with a knife. This is a painstaking process and will be easiest the sooner you do it. The root dries quickly, and the bark becomes very difficult to remove. It is important to add vegetable glycerin to this tincture to help the saponins and tannins coexist. Normally, they are enemies in solution and will precipitate out and form a dark goop at the bottom of the tincture.

Dosage: Take 5 to 10 drops 3 to 5 times a day. Best mixed with other tinctures.

5 ounces fresh red root bark
5 fluid ounces 190-proof alcohol
(95 percent), such as Everclear
4 fluid ounces water
1 fluid ounce vegetable glycerin

Put the bark into a clean 16-ounce jar and pour in the alcohol, water, and glycerin. Put the lid on and give it a good shake.

Label well, making sure to include the added vegetable glycerin (i.e., 50 percent alcohol, 10 percent glycerin).

Let sit in a cool, dark place, shaking occasionally, for 1 month. The tincture should start to turn red within the first day.

When it's ready to strain, use cheesecloth to strain out the chunks of root bark and return it to the original jar. Store in a cool, dark place for up to 5 years.

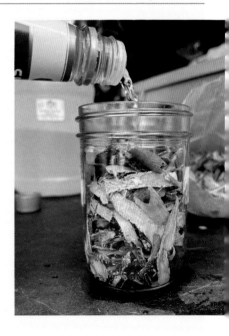

For medicine, you will use whatever part of the root is red or pink. Usually it is just the bark of the root that carries these pigments, but sometimes the inner wood is also pink or red. The bark can be quite difficult and time-consuming to remove, and it becomes more difficult to remove as the root dries, so remove it as soon as possible. Set aside some time at home for this task or out in the field with a pocketknife, and place a large drop cloth underneath. For this particular peeling job, use a sharp pocketknife, peeling toward the ground and away from your body. Slightly angle the knife, and peel the pink/red bark off, leaving the white woody inner part.

Some herbalists who want to avoid digging the whole bush (which kills the plant) favor using the bark of the branches instead. Other herbalists argue that only the root bark has the right constituents. I have had great success using a tincture of branch bark, though I can tell by the less-strong flavor that there are fewer of certain constituents in it. The branches *are* much easier to harvest, though. All you need to do is saw off a few at the base and peel the bark with a knife. This is best done in the spring, before blooming, or in the fall.

The flowers must be harvested when fresh, in June or July, depending on the elevation and the year. They have a very distinct scent that can be smelled on the breeze of a warm day. Beetles seem to love these flowers, so you may need to hunt for some with fewer beetles, or be ready to blow the beetles off. The leaves can be harvested any time of year, but are particularly nice in summer. I dry them and add them to blends for coughs and colds.

Medicinal Uses of Red Root

The root bark of red root is the most commonly used part of the plant in modern American herbalism. It is primarily a lymphatic herb, meaning that it facilitates the movement and processing of lymph. It can be used for tonsillitis, laryngitis, cystic breast tissue, and infections that involve swollen lymph nodes like strep. It is also used for spleen and liver enlargement and swelling. It is very drying and therefore best mixed with other herbs in a formula or in small doses (see Cautions). I combine it with echinacea, which also acts on the lymph.

Red root also relieves congestion in the liver. A congested liver can cause skin breakouts, aching joints, menstrual issues, and certain types of headaches.

Though you will not find it for sale in any herb store or written about in many books, red root flower has a strong history of use among Indigenous peoples all across North America. It is less astringent than the root bark and still contains saponins, making it a less potent but more palatable medicine. It is used similarly for infections and congestion. I combine it in a wild-crafted tea formula for coughs and colds with other herbs like elderberry, elderflower, pearly everlasting, yarrow, fir tips, and wild cherry bark.

Making Medicine with Red Root

A tincture of the fresh root bark of red root is the most classic preparation (see Tincture of Fresh Red Root Bark). It is important to add vegetable glycerin to this tincture because red root contains both tannins and saponins. When those two constituents exist together in solution, they react, and the tannins precipitate out and turn into a dark globular mass at the bottom of the tincture. Glycerin helps the tannins stay in solution.

If you are ever wondering if a plant contains saponins, simply put it in water in a jar and shake it up. If it has them, it will create foam much like soap! Red root flowers, leaves, and roots all contain saponins—if you rub the leaves in your hands with some water, they will foam up.

I dry the flowers and use them in tea, which I often combine with fir tips. The leaves can also be used in tea—both dried and toasted—but I am not a big fan of the flavor.

Cautions

The root bark of red root is very drying and astringent. To avoid dehydration, constipation, or other complications from taking strong astringents, add a moistening herb like licorice root. Also, take only small doses of this herb at a time: 5 drops when used alone, or 10 percent of a formula.

Rose

Rosa nutkana, R. rugosa, R. canina
Rosaceae (rose family)

How can you identify a rose? If it looks like a rose, and it smells like a rose, then it's a rose. And if it smells good, then it will make good medicine. There are two main species of wild rose that I like to harvest here in the Pacific Northwest. There are several other species as well, but they are less aromatic and less common than these two.

My favorite is rugosa rose (*Rosa rugosa*) because it creates the most flowers, the most petals, the best scent, and the largest, juiciest rose hips. It is not native to our area, but has naturalized in several places because of its vigorous growth habit. It is also planted in many parks and median strips because it is low maintenance. This rose blooms more when you harvest the flowers. However, it is nice to leave some of the flowers on the bush for the bees, who love roses dearly.

Nootka rose (*Rosa nutkana*) is native and is the most common rose in our area. It smells absolutely divine, though its flowers are much smaller and not as easy to harvest in large quantities. That said, there are areas in the drier microclimates around the Puget Sound that have nootka roses in such abundance that you can get quite a large bag and still leave flowers on the bush for the bees.

LEFT There are several varieties of rugosa rose, including this pretty white one. They all make great medicine. **RIGHT** Rose hips can persist into December and January, becoming winter forage for insects and animals.

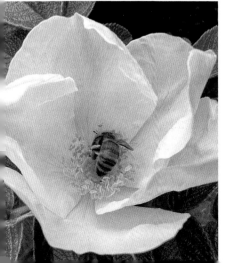
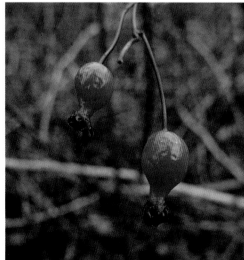

Rugosa rose
Rosa rugosa

Rose hip

Petal

Leaf

Stipules at the
base of the leaf →

Look for the sharp,
needle-like thorns.

Bud

Flowers

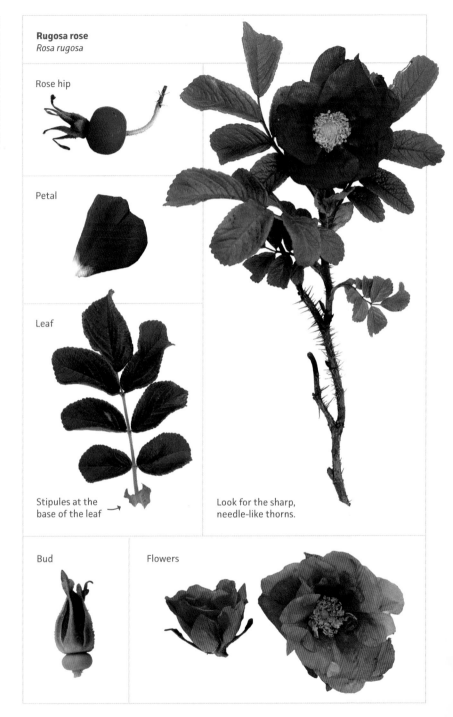

Several other species of wild roses have flowers and hips that are nice to harvest as well. Use taste and smell to shop your neighborhood plants. If you're looking for a good candidate for your garden, there are also some really nice roses that are bred for their scent, the most famous being damask rose (*Rosa damascena*), which grows nicely here when tended in a garden.

Harvesting Rose

Roses are typically in their best bloom in May and early June. Some species will continue blooming, but typically it gets too hot and too dry for them in our area.

Harvest the petals on a dry day just after they have opened, when they are the most fragrant. If you take all the petals but one, the bees can still find the flower and pollinate it. When you get home, either lay the petals out to dry immediately or make your medicine while they're fresh. You can store them in the fridge for a day or two, but you'll lose some of the delicate aromatics.

The hips ripen at various times in the fall. Rugosa rose ripens first and has soft hips that rot quickly. Other roses, like dog rose (*Rosa canina*), ripen in late November and will stay on the bush all winter. To determine whether a rose hip is ripe, look for orange flesh and taste to see if it's sweeter rather than more sour and astringent. Keep in mind that rose hips have hairs around the seeds that are highly irritating to the gastrointestinal tract. They are so irritating that they used to be made into itching powder and sold at the joke shop. Herbalists get around this by removing the hairs by hand or straining the tea really well.

LEFT Harvesting nootka rose blossoms in a community garden **RIGHT** It is hard to harvest the flowers without disturbing the bees, who absolutely adore rose.

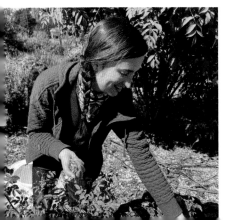
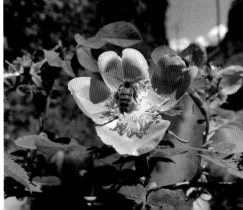

Nootka rose
Rosa nutkana

Rose hip

A rose gall forms when a wasp lays eggs in the stem of the plant. As the wasps mature inside, the plant is stimulated to create this protective casing.

New growth has very few thorns.

A progression from bud to flower

Five-petaled flowers

The hip already beginning to form

Medicinal Uses of Rose

Rose petals are used in cosmetics for their anti-inflammatory, anti-scarring, tissue-regenerative, astringent, and antioxidant actions. Rose can be used for acne, scarring, eczema, psoriasis, aging skin, rashes, and itching. I spray rose water (which is actually rose hydrosol) on my face before I put on my face oil. It soaks into my skin under the oil and hydrates nicely. You can also add powdered rose petals to a face mask. Try mixing the powder with honey and applying the paste to your face.

Taken internally, roses have an affinity for the liver, the blood vessels, and the heart. Rose petal tea helps lessen menstrual symptoms like cramps and mood swings when they are caused by liver or blood stagnation. I combine rose with St. John's wort for this purpose. Rose petals are very astringent. In fact, a cold tea of rose petals can be used to reduce hemorrhage and to help stop a bleeding wound. A strong rose tea can also be used as a rinse for an itchy scalp.

Rose petals are frequently added to formulas for depression along with herbs like lemon balm, albizzia, and St. John's wort. Similarly, rose is in most aphrodisiac formulas because of its ability to relax and open the heart.

Hawthorn and rose are a great duo for strengthening the heart and blood vessels. Both of these herbs are rich in compounds that support the physical heart and are also heavily associated with the energetic heart—more specifically love and passion.

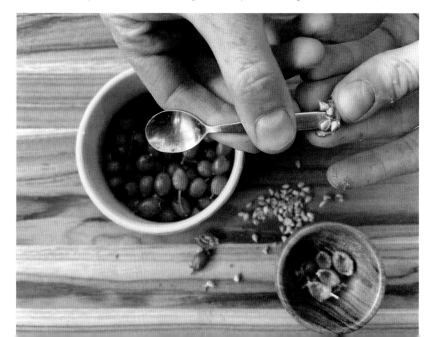

Removing the seeds and hairs from rose hips using the back of a spoon

Rose hips are primarily known for their high vitamin C content, evidenced by their very sour taste. They are also high in flavonoids, much like the petals. Both vitamin C and flavonoids are different types of antioxidants, so many of the uses of rose hips revolve around that. Drinking rose hip tea is thought to support the immune system and to slow aging.

Making Medicine with Rose

To make tea from rose petals, steep 1 to 2 tablespoons of dried petals in a covered mug of hot water for 10 minutes, then strain and drink. The tea is a bit astringent for me to drink straight, so I add a little honey. That said, I typically mix it with other things, such as chamomile, hibiscus, or holy basil.

A tincture of rose petals should be made with a slightly higher alcohol content than other tinctures. I use 60 percent because it's high enough to capture the aromatic compounds but not high enough to burn your mouth (see Tincture Ratio Chart). You can also make a rose glycerite, which tastes absolutely delicious and isn't as drying. I don't include instructions on how to make a glycerite in this book, but you can find instructions online.

Rose petal infused honey is my favorite preparation of rose (see Rose Infused Honey). Speaking of sweet, rosy things, you can also make rose cordial with alcohol and sugar, or you can make rose petal conserve or jam.

Rose hips can be boiled in water for tea or made into jam or a simple syrup. You can also make a rose hip tincture (see Tincture Ratio Chart). There are a lot of Eastern European grocery stores in my area that sell rose hip products, including bottles of rose hip beverages sweetened with sugar.

Cautions

Rose petals can be very drying and astringent when taken internally. Excessive use may cause constipation or dehydration.

ROSE INFUSED HONEY   *Makes about 2 cups of honey*

This sweet, floral honey is my favorite of all infused honeys, and I make at least one batch every year. I eat it on pancakes, yogurt, and almond cake, and use it in tea. It's best to use a very neutral-tasting honey for this project, like clover honey, as the delicate rose flavor can get lost among stronger flavors.

2 cups fresh, whole rose petals, enough
    to fill a 16-ounce jar
About 2 cups honey

Add the rose petals to a clean 16-ounce jar, tamping them down a little with clean hands. Pour honey over the top, pausing to let the honey sink down into the jar before adding more. The level of the honey should meet the level of the rose petals in the jar.

    Prepare a hot water bath by adding a few inches of water to a medium saucepan and setting it on the stove, or add the water to a slow cooker. Place the jar in the saucepan or slow cooker. I always put the jar in before turning on the heat, as the difference in temperature can crack the bottom of the jar if you put it in when the water is hot. Add a bit of water if needed to ensure the level of the water is equal to the level of the honey in the jar.

    With the uncovered jar sitting in the water bath, turn the heat on as low as possible. Leave the jar to sit in the water bath for 1 or 2 hours. Rose is very delicate, so I heat it for less time than I might for other herbs.

    When finished, strain through a fine-mesh strainer into a new 16-ounce jar while the honey is still warm enough to pour easily. Though it's not strictly necessary, I sometimes store it in the fridge because a lot of water has been introduced from the petals, which can sometimes be enough to result in fermentation.

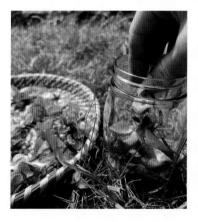
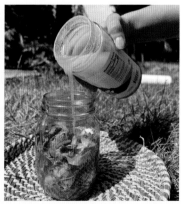

Spruce

Picea sitchensis, P. engelmannii
Pinaceae (pine family)

We have two main species of native spruce in the Pacific Northwest: Sitka spruce (*Picea sitchensis*) and Engelmann spruce (*Picea engelmannii*). There are several ornamental species that are planted in gardens, parks, and public landscapes that are good for harvest as well.

Developing
Sitka spruce
cones

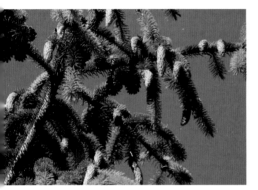

Sitka spruce is the most common spruce found here, thriving along the Pacific coast from Alaska to Northern California. You will find it in coastal forests along the Pacific Ocean and Puget Sound. These coastal spruce forests are absolutely amazing, with an understory filled with red elderberry bushes larger than you've ever seen, sword fern, salmonberry, false lily of the valley, devil's club, and red huckleberry. In spruce forests, the fire interval—the number of years, on average, between fires—is very high, with fire expected between every 150 to 350 years or more. Unlike its cousin ponderosa pine, Sitka spruce is not well adapted to fire, with its thin bark and roots close to the surface. Sitka spruce is a tree of the classic wet, quiet, and foggy forests of the Pacific coast that soothe my soul.

Sitka spruce is an important tree to many of the Northwest Coast Native groups and is used for construction, basketry, medicine, and more.

Identifying spruce is fairly easy—most species have extremely sharp needles that stab you when grabbed. Here's a mnemonic that my students and I made up to remember the pine-family trees:

Spruce stabs,
pine has packets,
fir is fragrant,
larch loses its needles,
hemlock hangs,
Douglas-fir doesn't fit.

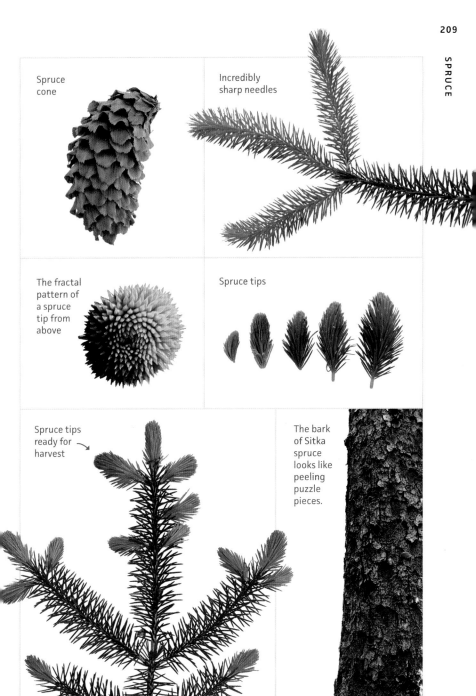

Spruce cone

Incredibly sharp needles

The fractal pattern of a spruce tip from above

Spruce tips

Spruce tips ready for harvest

The bark of Sitka spruce looks like peeling puzzle pieces.

Pine needles are grouped into "packets," formally called fascicles. The tops of hemlock trees are soft and thus they bend and hang downward. And Douglas-fir, despite having *fir* in the name, is not part of the fir genus. Thus it "doesn't fit."

Harvesting Spruce

Spruce tips can be harvested from April to June. The tips are the new vegetative growth for the entire year, emerging as a tender lime-green shoot. These shoots are aromatic, somewhat sweet, and much less astringent than the older needles and branches.

I typically harvest from ornamental varieties that grow in parks, partially because the branches are much lower and reachable. Test the medicinal quality of an unknown spruce variety by squishing and smelling the tips and needles to see how aromatic they are before you harvest. You can even nibble on one to see if it's got a nice flavor.

The needles can also be harvested later in the year and even in the winter. Wear gloves for harvesting as the mature needles of some species are so sharp they can draw blood.

LEFT Harvesting the tips from an ornamental spruce tree in a local park **RIGHT** Resin on a fallen spruce tree in a park—a great opportunity to harvest!

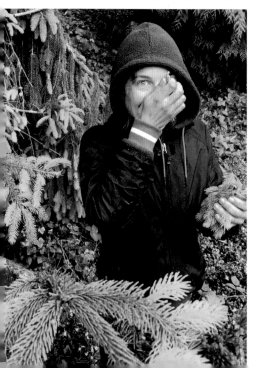 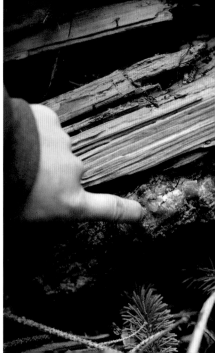

From the trunk of the tree, you can also harvest spruce resin, which drips from places where the bark has been broken or cut. Don't pick the resin out of the gash itself, as the tree is using the resin there to seal itself from diseases, much like a human scab. Instead, pick resin that has dripped from the wound down the side of the tree. The drier, harder bits are less sticky and easier to work with.

Medicinal Uses of Spruce

The medicinal uses of spruce do not diverge greatly from other pine-family trees. Spruce tips and needles are expectorant, very high in vitamin C, antibacterial, antifungal, and antioxidant. They are a great choice for winter respiratory wellness and also for preventing and combating coughs and colds.

The resin of spruce is a traditional remedy for infected wounds, sores, ulcers, and burns. Not only is it antibacterial, but it also helps the skin heal faster, making resin a great thing to have in your first aid kit for cuts. Because it is oil soluble, the resin is commonly prepared in an oil-based ointment or salve (see Pine Resin Salve).

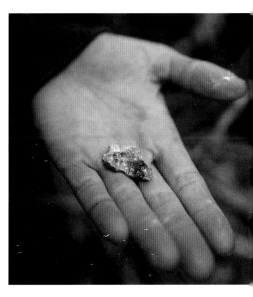

A chunk of spruce resin ready to take home and dissolve in oil

The resin can also be applied directly to the skin to help pull out a splinter: Add a bit of resin to the site of the splinter, put an adhesive bandage over it, and let it do its work overnight. Take the bandage off the next day, and hopefully the resin will have pulled the splinter to the surface enough to remove it. This remedy is Scandinavian, where there is a strong tradition of using spruce and other pine-family trees for medicine.

In Scandinavia and among the Native groups of the Pacific Northwest, spruce resin has been used as a chewing gum. Sometimes when I am hiking, I like to take a drop of resin and adhere it to the roof of my mouth, where it stays for most of the day and provides a fresh, piney flavor. Definitely good for a sore throat!

Making Medicine with Spruce

Spruce tips are prepared most often in culinary creations because of their nice flavor, with notes of tropical fruit and lavender. People make infused sugar, syrups, infused honey, tea, bitters, and even things like panna cotta. In some cases, the tips are infused and then strained out, and in others, they are ground into the final preparation (like spruce-tip infused sugar).

A cold or hot infusion is the most typical way that herbalists prepare the tips for medicine. To make a cold infusion of spruce tips, put a few handfuls at the bottom of a 32-ounce mason jar,

---

SPRUCE TIP OXYMEL　　　　　　　　　　　　　　*Makes 1 to 1½ cups*

An oxymel is a mix of honey and vinegar infused with a plant. I love to make oxymels of spruce, fir, and Douglas-fir. You can mix it with sparkling water, ice, and a lemon wedge for a lemony, refreshing non-alcoholic beverage. Spruce oxymel is also a great winter lung tonic and can be taken by the teaspoonful. Chopping the tips first will expose some of the inside of the needles and ensure you get a better extraction.

---

2 cups chopped spruce tips
¾ cup honey
¾ cup apple cider vinegar

Fill a clean 16-ounce jar with spruce tips up to the top, packing them loosely with your fingers.

Pour the honey and vinegar into a large measuring cup or medium bowl and mix together with a whisk until the honey is dissolved. Pour the honey and vinegar mixture into the jar until it reaches the level of the tips. Store any extra honey-vinegar mixture in the fridge for later use.

Use a plastic lid to seal the jar and shake it for a bit.

Let sit in a cool, dark place for 2 weeks.

Strain using a piece of cheesecloth, squeezing with your hands to get everything out.

Store the oxymel in a 16-ounce jar or bottle in the fridge for up to 1 year.

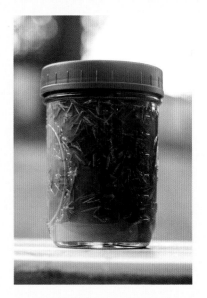

Avoid metal lids when working with vinegar, as the acidic solution corrodes the metal.

fill it with water, and let it sit in the fridge overnight. The result is a very refreshing flavored water. Mature spruce needles can also be used for the cold infusion, though it's best if you remove the stems and crush the needles a bit before infusing. Hot infusions should be made exclusively from the tips and new growth (the heat pulls out undesirable compounds from older growth that make the tea taste astringent and camphor-like). Add about ¼ cup of tips to 8 ounces of boiling water. Cover and let sit for 7 to 10 minutes, and then strain and drink. It's nice with honey, and even better with spruce-tip infused honey.

Avoid using alcohol in any spruce-needle preparation as it draws out some of the astringent and camphor compounds that can make it taste like turpentine. Honey, however, seems to be able to extract the tasty compounds from spruce and avoid the yucky ones. To make an infused honey, loosely pack a jar with chopped needles, pour honey over the top, then put it in a hot water bath for 4 to 8 hours (see the Rose Infused Honey recipe for details). Strain the mixture through a fine-mesh strainer to remove the tips. I find spruce-needle honey to be stronger and more delicious than spruce-tip honey.

A lot of good flavor is lost when you dry spruce tips and needles, so try to use them fresh. That said, I do sometimes dry some tips for hot infusions later in the season.

Cautions

Spruce resin should not be taken internally in large doses, and use caution when taking even small amounts internally. Resin from pine-family trees can cause kidney damage when taken internally. Historical accounts refer to pine resin being used internally, but that does not necessarily mean it is safe. Do not take pine bark internally for long periods or in large doses.

St. John's Wort

Hypericum perforatum
Hypericaceae (St. John's wort family)

This is a non-native plant that's considered a Class C noxious weed in Washington State, so no one will begrudge you harvesting it. The reason for this classification is that it can be fatal to cows if they eat too much, and it has been particularly pervasive on ranchlands in Washington. St. John's wort has been such a concern for ranchers that it was the victim of the first insect biocontrol agent in the United States, the Klamathweed beetle (Klamathweed is another name for St. John's wort). The beetle was introduced as a specialized pest to feed on St. John's wort and reduce its population. You will likely see it while you're out harvesting!

A tiny Klamath-weed beetle happily feeding on a St. John's wort plant

Note that there are a few species of ornamental St. John's wort in the *Hypericum* genus that are not the medicinal variety. The species featured in this book—*Hypericum perforatum*—is the one you want. Look for the leaf perforations and check for the red squish from the buds if you are unsure (see photos).

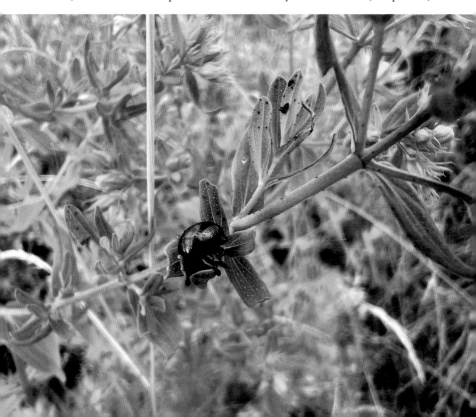

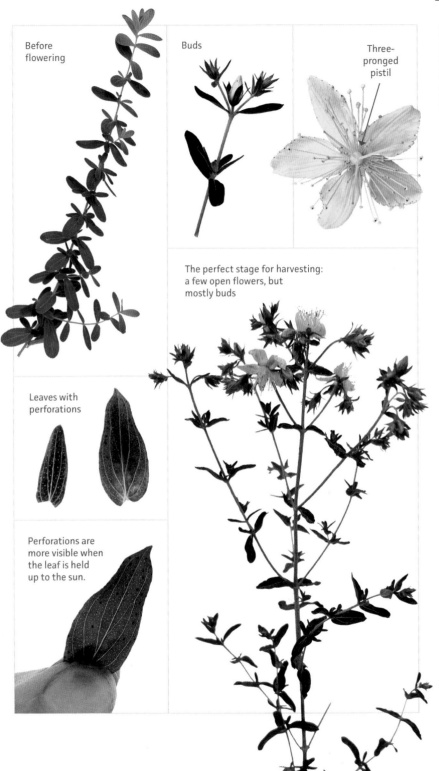

Before flowering

Buds

Three-pronged pistil

The perfect stage for harvesting: a few open flowers, but mostly buds

Leaves with perforations

Perforations are more visible when the leaf is held up to the sun.

Harvesting St. John's Wort

Harvest the flowering tops ideally when most of the flowers are still in bud, with just a few open. The buds should be fat and yellow and exude a good amount of red when squished. St. John's wort blooms around the summer solstice (on or about June 21) at sea level in the Puget Sound region. At higher elevations (such as in the Cascades), it typically blooms in late July and sometimes even in August.

St. John's wort prefers open areas, especially where the soil is rocky and poor, such as a prairie, seasonal riverbed, or roadsides. I often see it within 10 feet of highways and forest service roads but not beyond. This is annoying for a harvester who shouldn't harvest right next to a main road due to pollution. The best harvest spots I have found are along old forest service roads that no longer see traffic and get a lot of sun. It may be abundant next to powerline trails, but be aware that the Department of Transportation often sprays pesticides to keep weeds at bay in these areas.

To pick, you can either snip off the top with clippers or use your fingers like a fork to scrape the buds off the tops. Make your medicine immediately upon arriving home as the buds lose their potency as they dry. Even so, I do dry some to add to tea blends and find it still quite effective.

LEFT Harvesting flowers using the "fork fingers" method RIGHT The buds, when squashed, produce a dark-red color.

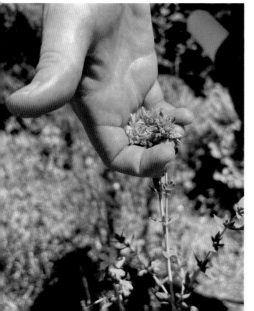
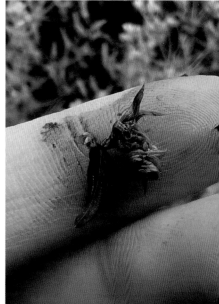

You can easily introduce St. John's wort into your garden by digging it up at any stage of growth (though best in spring) and planting it in your yard in a sunny spot. Under your care, it will likely thrive and become a hearty patch.

Medicinal Uses of St. John's Wort

Before using St. John's wort internally, be aware that it interacts with a huge number of medications, so care should be taken to check on the herb-and-drug interactions (see Cautions). I advise folks who are taking pharmaceuticals to steer clear of St. John's wort.

That said, St. John's wort is one of the most useful and effective herbs in my apothecary, so let's talk about the details. It is astringent (dries and tightens tissue), vulnerary (heals wounds), diuretic (makes you pee), antimicrobial (kills bacteria and other microbes), and analgesic (relieves pain).

St. John's wort also stimulates liver function quite effectively. An out-of-balance liver is like an out-of-tune guitar string that makes a jarring, cantankerous noise when plucked. In a similar energetic fashion, when the liver is out of balance, the feeling in the body will become cantankerous. Anger and irritability can be caused by a disharmonious liver. St. John's wort can help the liver come back into balance and can sometimes bring down a temper!

Hormonal fluctuations can bring disharmony to the liver, which is a typical cause of PMS. St. John's wort is my favorite remedy for that hurricane-like hormonal frustration; it can reduce my acute irritation miraculously by just taking a dropperful or two of the tincture when the feeling comes. A disharmony in the liver can also cause stomach issues, reflux among them. So it is not surprising that St. John's wort also eases reflux caused by stress.

St. John's wort is primarily known for its effectiveness for depression, which has been studied and widely proclaimed. Building off the liver/guitar-string metaphor, it will be most effective for folks with tense, angsty, frustrated, and moody depression. This is a depression of a stagnant liver, which this herb helps relieve by clearing it out and opening up the flow. For this, it is usually used internally as a tincture. Dose at about 1 to 2 dropperfuls as needed for acute events, or 1 dropperful 2 to 3 times a day for depression.

St. John's wort is also touted as a nerve tonic and nerve pain reliever. I have seen it used externally for gout pain with success, for example. Use it on sciatica, back pain, and areas with nerve damage. For these, it can be used topically as an oil and internally as a tea or tincture. Applying often and consistently is a good way to ensure success—make sure you're using a potent product. That goes for all topical remedies.

Using St. John's wort as a wound healer goes all the way back to ancient Greece, where wounds were cleaned with the infused oil. A decoction used as a wound wash would also be a great application. It can be used for bruises and blunt force trauma as well, and is often combined with arnica for this purpose.

ST. JOHN'S WORT OIL   *Makes 1½ cups*

Any preparation using this amazing plant has to be made with fresh plant material in order to extract the active medicinal constituent, hypericin, and the quality of the harvest is key: Use only the best flowering tops and buds to make the oil. In addition, the most potent oil is made from plants that received the most sun, which means that harvesting east of the Cascades is ideal. After harvesting the buds and fresh flowering tops, leave the plant to wilt for a few hours. Carefully pick out all the insects and remove them during this time.

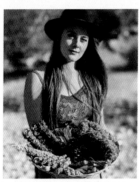

To make the oil, you will use heat to gently evaporate the water content out of the plant material while extracting the hypericin into the oil. Two methods are outlined here: using the sun and a hot water bath. For the carrier oil, I like to use olive oil or meadowfoam seed oil because of their shelf life and healing properties. This recipe was contributed by Cricket McCormick, who is passionate about natural healing. Cricket has traveled to many countries and studied different ancient healing modalities at their source.

Cricket McCormick

Dosage: Apply to the affected area of skin 2 to 3 times a day.

2 cups fresh St. John's wort flowers and buds
1½ cups organic extra-virgin olive oil or other
    oil of your choosing, plus more as needed

Loosely pack the flowers and buds into a clean, dry 16-ounce jar, filling it about three-quarters full.

Pour the oil into the jar to about ¼ inch from the top. Use a utensil to push the plant matter down and allow air bubbles to come up.

St. John's wort is also excellent at cleaning the walls of the bladder in cases of chronic infections, irritability, and cloudy urine. It is astringent, a wound healer, and antimicrobial. Studies suggest uses for treating incontinence and interstitial cystitis. I combine it in a tea with corn silk and lemon verbena for bladder irritability and urinary frequency.

Making Medicine with St. John's Wort

Because one of the important medicinal constituents degrades during the drying process, St. John's wort preparations are

Cut squares of cheesecloth to fit over the top of the jar and secure the cloth by screwing the rim of the canning lid onto the jar. This opening will allow the moisture in the plant matter to evaporate.

For the solar-infusion method, the sun needs to be shining. Place your jar in a paper bag and set it out in the warm sun each day for a few hours at a time, until the oil becomes saturated with the reddish/burgundy color. This process can take to 4 to 6 weeks.

If a solar infusion is not possible, then use the hot-water-bath method. Place the jar in a slow cooker filled with water (or other homemade hot-water-bath setup). The water should reach the level of the oil in the jar. Do not allow the cheesecloth on top of the jar to touch the water or it could draw more moisture into the oil.

Put the slow cooker on the lowest setting, and test the temperature of the water periodically to make sure it does not exceed 120°F. Slow cookers with a "warm" setting are ideal for this. You will likely need to turn the slow cooker on and off to keep it from overheating. If this is the case for your slow cooker, turn it off during the night, and then on again in the morning. If the plant material becomes crispy, it has been overheated. Let the jar sit in the water of the slow cooker for 48 hours, or until the oil is a deep red.

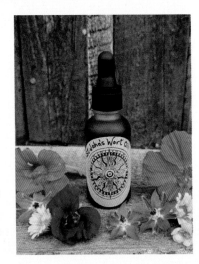

Once finished, strain the plant material using cheesecloth and put the oil in a clean, dry 16-ounce jar.

After a day, the sediment from the oil will settle. Decant the oil, and discard the sediment. This extra step will help make the oil last longer. Bottle and keep in a cool, dark place for up to 1 year. You may also store it in the fridge to make it last longer, but that is not required.

made with very fresh plant material. I do use the dried flowering tops in tea blends, though in dried form they lack some of the medicinal action.

The best way to capture the medicine of the fresh buds is to make a tincture, which should be blood red in color (see Tincture Ratio Chart). I blend the buds with the alcohol to increase extraction.

An infused oil of the buds is also commonly used and should be deep red in color (see St. John's Wort Oil).

Cautions

There are several cautions for St. John's wort, the most notable being that it has many serious interactions with medications. It is not within the scope of this book to discuss specific herb-and-drug interactions, so please research it for yourself. As stated, I generally discourage people who take pharmaceuticals from using St. John's wort.

Another caution is that it can theoretically cause photosensitivity of the skin for some people when consumed internally or applied externally. I have never heard of this happening, but it is taught as a possibility and so I pass that on here.

I have seen St. John's wort awaken anger in people, which is an indication of its role as a liver cleanser. Old anger—as well as old toxins—hang out in the liver, which St. John's wort releases. This can cause detox reactions and emotional reactions from its use. If you choose to use St. John's wort, I suggest the low-and-slow approach. For example, 5 drops of St. John's wort tincture per day for 3 months.

Usnea

Usnea spp.
Parmeliaceae (usnea family)

Usnea is also known as old man's beard or beard lichen. Herbalists more commonly call it usnea, so that is the name I use here. *Usnea* is also the name of the genus this lichen is in, so if it is written in italics, I am referring to the genus.

Usnea is not a plant; it is a lichen. A lichen is two organisms working together: a fungus and an algae or cyanobacteria. The fungus provides structure and water retention, and the algae or cyanobacteria provides the food through photosynthesis. Unlike mushrooms and plants, lichens don't have roots. They do have a structure that holds them to their substrate, like a branch or rock, where they live.

Lichens have a lot of important roles in ecosystems. They fix nitrogen from the air into usable nitrogen for the forest. This is quite important, especially somewhere with nitrogen-poor soils like the Pacific Northwest. Lichens also erode rock to make soil, which is important after something like a volcanic eruption that annihilates all life and leaves nothing but rock. Also, lichens can stabilize parts of sand dunes and pioneer the way for other species to grow. Lichens also provide food and habitat for creatures such as deer. Humans can eat it too, though most species cause gastrointestinal (GI) distress if not prepared properly. While it's not necessarily my food of choice, lichen has been a winter famine food in places like Sweden and Norway.

Something else of note about lichen is that most of them are very sensitive to air pollution, so if there's a lot of lichens around, you know that there's clean air. In fact, researchers monitor lichens as an indicator of climate change and air pollution.

There are various species of usnea that all have different preferences. Look out into a winter swamp, and you might see the vine maples and red osier dogwoods covered in the pastel-green fuzz of usnea. In a beautiful coniferous rainforest, you might see the famously long *Usnea longissima* hanging like a garland. Or on the branches of an old apple

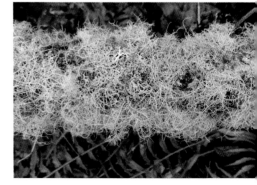

Usnea mixed with other lichens on a red alder branch

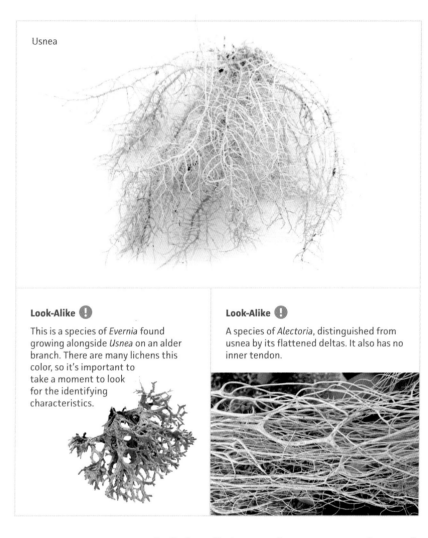

Usnea

Look-Alike ⚠️

This is a species of *Evernia* found growing alongside *Usnea* on an alder branch. There are many lichens this color, so it's important to take a moment to look for the identifying characteristics.

Look-Alike ⚠️

A species of *Alectoria*, distinguished from usnea by its flattened deltas. It also has no inner tendon.

tree, you might find small clusters of usnea growing along with *Evernia* spp. and a party of other lichens.

Several genuses of lichens can be mistaken for usnea, most notably *Ramalina* spp., *Evernia* spp., and *Alectoria* spp. These lichens are similar in color, structure, and habitat but will not pass the tendon test. *Ramalina* has flat lobes and no central tendon, and *Evernia* is also flat, but has a lighter-colored underside. *Alectoria* is the most similar to usnea. The easiest way to tell *Alectoria* and *Usnea* apart is the tendon test, but also note *Alectoria* will be flattened at the intersections of branches, and *Usnea* species will always be cylindrical.

Usnea always grows on trees. Alder especially gets covered in it. There are a few branched lichens that are similar in color and shape, but they grow on the ground, like certain species of *Cladonia*.

The only toxic species of lichen I know of in Washington is *Letharia* spp., known as "wolf lichen." It is bright yellow and grows only on the east side of the Cascades.

Note that Spanish moss (*Tillandsia usneoides*), which resembles usnea in its color and growth habit, is not a lichen at all, but a flowering plant in the bromeliad family.

Some *Usnea* species are abundant (like the ones that grow on alder trees), but *Usnea longissima* is currently threatened due to air pollution, overharvesting (by the floral industry), and habitat loss from logging. It prefers old-growth or late-succession (i.e., logged a long time ago) conifer forests and loves north- or northeast-facing hillsides that see a lot of fog. In Washington State, I think of those places with giant Douglas-fir and hemlock trees that constantly seem to have a cloud hugging a hillside, where everything is wet and green.

Harvesting Usnea

I like to harvest usnea after a winter storm, from fallen red alder branches or from the ground. The lichen is typically still alive when you harvest it, but check for rot: it will look like it is melting into white or brown goo. I collect quite a bit to make a tincture, as it dries and loses a lot of weight.

LEFT Harvesting usnea in January after a windstorm **RIGHT** Confirming my ID by using the tendon test. The outer skin breaks, revealing a rubbery white tendon within.

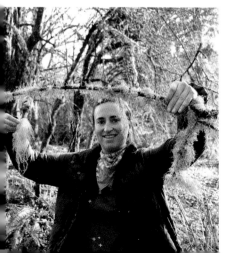
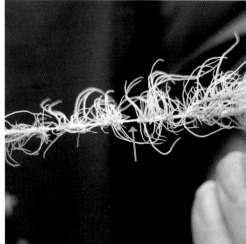

The best usnea patches I have found are in mature red alder forests, where the alders are reaching their terminal age and they are starting to get brittle and fall over in storms. Alder trees are the first step of building a forest, like the first person to show up to a party. They stabilize the soil and fix nitrogen. After about sixty years, they die and make way for the next species in the succession, which are typically maple and Douglas-fir. When you look up into one of these forests of alders, the bark is often spotted with various lichen, fungi, and mosses, and you'll be able to see the trees' cones and catkins dangling like ornaments. Especially if you're in a spot that's moist and north facing, you should see thick tufts of usnea hanging off the trees everywhere.

Usnea, unlike its look-alikes, has a rubber band–like skeleton inside the green outer skin. To confirm that what you have plucked is usnea, tug gently on one of the central strings of the lichen: The outer skin should break and reveal the rubber band–like skeleton stretching out inside. This is called the "tendon test" because the white filament inside resembles a tendon. Also, the structure of usnea is always cylindrical like a branch and never flattened like a leaf.

To be a good steward of *Usnea longissima* and other usnea species, carry it from where it's fallen on the ground and drape it onto a new branch. Many lichens can reproduce asexually by breaking off their original home and falling onto another branch. Lichens apparently struggle to spread very far by themselves, but thrive on humans propagating them in new areas.

Deer and other creatures sometimes eat usnea and other lichens in the winter. It's not a preferred food choice, but they seek it out when not much else is around. It's important to leave lichen on the ground when there is snow, as it can be the only food available to certain creatures.

Medicinal Uses of Usnea

Usnea has two major actions: antimicrobial and immunomodulation. An immunomodulator helps regulate the immune system to the correct level of response, rather than simply suppressing or stimulating the immune system.

The antimicrobial action of usnea is what it is most known for. (The word *microbe* applies to bacteria, fungi, viruses, and usually protozoa.) It is very effective against gram-positive

USNEA DOUBLE EXTRACT

Makes about 20 ounces

A double extract is a type of tincture that uses both hot water and alcohol to extract the constituents. Because usnea has alcohol-soluble constituents (usnic acid) and hot-water-soluble constituents (polysaccharides), this method is necessary to make an effective tincture. There are several slightly different methods to make a double extract. In this recipe, we boil the lichen in water and then add alcohol to the slurry. Note that this is a more advanced medicine-making technique.

Dosage: Take 30 to 60 drops 3 to 5 times a day.

2 ounces dried usnea lichen
20 fluid ounces water
10 fluid ounces 190-proof alcohol
  (95 percent), such as Everclear

Grind the lichen or chop very finely to expose the white inner cortex, which is the part that contains the polysaccharides.

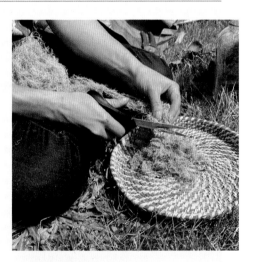

Combine the lichen and water in a large pot and bring to a boil over high heat. Reduce to low and simmer for 1 hour with the lid off. During this time, half of the water should evaporate, leaving you with 10 fluid ounces of liquid. If the stove is too hot, it may evaporate too quickly, so watch carefully.

The liquid should be cloudy, and the usnea will be gloppy. Let this mixture cool enough to pour into a 32-ounce heat-proof jar.

Add the alcohol when the mixture is warm but not hot. Put the lid on.

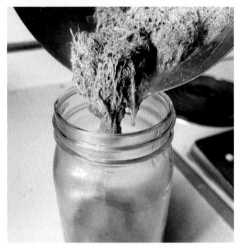

Wait about an hour for it to cool, then give it a shake. If you shake it too soon, or if the lid isn't on tight, it can spurt out of the jar due to the pressure from the heat.

Let sit in a cool, dark place for 4 weeks and then strain. Store in a clean glass jar in a cool, dark place for up to 5 years.

bacteria, which includes infection-causing bacteria such as staphylococcus, streptococcus, and tuberculosis. It is not as effective against gram-negative bacteria but has been found somewhat useful against some important infection-causing gram-negative bacteria, such as *Helicobacter pylori*, *E. coli*, *Yersinia enterocolitica*, and *Proteus mirabilis*. To simplify the point, usnea tincture is used for respiratory infections (lung and sinus), throat infections, GI infections, and urinary tract infections. It can also be used for skin infections like impetigo: wash sores twice a day with soap and apply the tincture to the affected areas.

It is considered to be effective against some viruses: herpes simplex, polyomavirus, Junín virus, Tacaribe virus, and Epstein-Barr. It's also effective against *Trichomonas* (protozoa) and many kinds of fungi, including some *Candida* species.

Making Medicine with Usnea

The antimicrobial action is rooted in the outer skin of the lichen and comes primarily from a compound called usnic acid, which is alcohol soluble. The immunomodulation action is derived from polysaccharides that come from the inner white tendon, which is hot-water soluble (meaning that to extract it, you have to boil it in water). These two compounds have different extraction needs; to make an effective usnea tincture, you need to make a double extract, also known as an alcohol-and-hot-water extract (see Usnea Double Extract). This preparation is a hybrid of a tincture and a decoction, which extracts both water-soluble polysaccharides and alcohol-soluble usnic acid.

You can also prepare a decoction of usnea as a wound soak or an immune-boosting drink, but it will not contain as many antimicrobial compounds.

Cautions

Don't use usnea internally during pregnancy. Usnea and other lichen tinctures can cause GI irritation in large doses, so it's best to take with about a half ounce of water.

Uva Ursi

Arctostaphylos nevadensis, A. uva-ursi
Ericaceae (heath family)

Uva ursi has been used by North American Indigenous cultures and Northern European cultures for many centuries. In Europe, the plant is more commonly known as bearberry, a name that alludes to how much bears love this berry. In America, it is more commonly known by the Algonquin name kinnikinnick, which means "smoking mixture." It is used in a ceremonial smoking blend by many Native groups in the northern US and in Canada.

There are two very similar species of *Arctostaphylos* growing in the Cascades that are quite hard to tell apart, but luckily, they're medicinally interchangeable. You'll find the more known *Arctostaphylos uva-ursi* all over the Pacific Northwest, including in the dry slopes above the Puget Sound, dry coniferous forests (especially with ponderosa pine), drought-tolerant landscaping, and parking lot median strips. Its close look-alike, *Arctostaphylos nevadensis*, is found only at middle-to-high elevations in the Cascades and has whiter flowers.

LEFT The urn-shaped flowers of uva ursi in full bloom **RIGHT** A ripe uva ursi berry

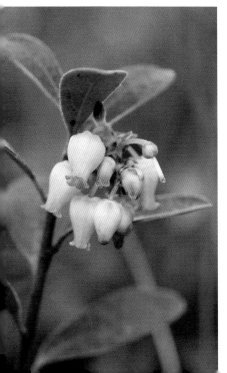
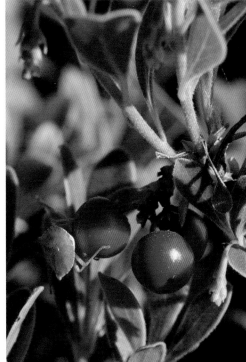

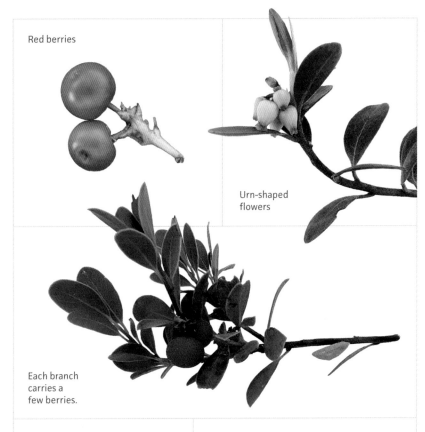

Red berries

Urn-shaped flowers

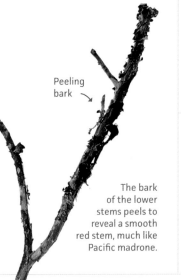

Each branch carries a few berries.

Peeling bark

The bark of the lower stems peels to reveal a smooth red stem, much like Pacific madrone.

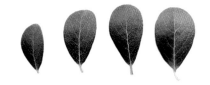

Leaves have round tips and smooth margins.

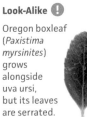

Look-Alike ⚠

Oregon boxleaf (*Paxistima myrsinites*) grows alongside uva ursi, but its leaves are serrated.

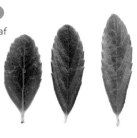

Harvesting Uva Ursi

Gather the leaves in September and October. Harvest where this plant is growing abundantly in thick mats along the ground, distributing your harvest so it doesn't look like you hacked a hole in the middle of the patch. Select whole stems and snip them off with scissors. Harvest the greenest leaves with the least signs of insect predation and fungal infection.

Make sure the weather is warm when you dry the leaves to prevent mold from growing. You could leave them outside in a large paper grocery bag tipped on its side on a warm sunny day, making sure the sun doesn't touch the leaves directly.

Fall is also when the small red berries are ripe. The berries are edible and can be eaten raw or cooked. They don't taste like much, so they are more of a survival food than a delightful gourmet berry.

Medicinal Uses of Uva Ursi

Uva ursi is astringent (dries and tightens tissues), antibacterial, soothing to inflamed tissue, and stimulating to the kidneys.

It is most commonly used for treating urinary tract infections. Because the astringent nature of uva ursi can irritate the stomach (see Cautions), herbalists often combine it with marshmallow root or another demulcent to counteract the astringency. Uva ursi is only effective for a urinary tract infection if the urine is alkaline. You can purchase pH strips to test

LEFT Snip off the newer growth on the ends. Select leaves that are clean and relatively untouched by insects and lichen. **RIGHT** Harvesting can be slow if you're being picky!

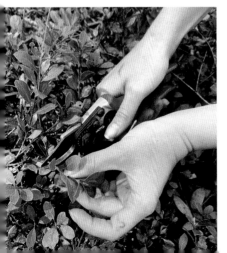
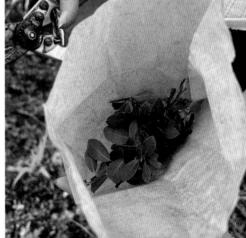

URINARY TRACT TEA   *Makes 1.5 ounces loose-leaf tea*

Make a quart of this tea and sip it throughout the day. The corn silk called for in this recipe is indeed the silk that comes from fresh corn. You can buy it dried, or you can pull it off fresh and dry it yourself. Corn silk tea tastes sweet and soothes inflammation in the bladder.

Dosage: Use ⅓ cup per quart of water. Infuse for 10 minutes, covered. Drink 1 to 2 cups a day.

1 ounce dried uva ursi leaf
1 ounce dried marshmallow root
0.5 ounce dried corn silk

Combine all ingredients in a medium bowl and mix well.
 Store in a jar for up to 2 years.

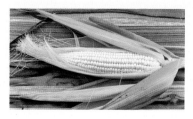

your urine at home. Uva ursi is most effective against *E. coli* bacteria, so urinary tract infections involving other bacteria may not respond to this plant. For those infections, try usnea lichen and Oregon grape.

The antibacterial action of this plant is associated with the compound arbutin. It is excreted through the kidneys and not through the large intestine, making it particularly effective for the urinary tract. Arbutin gets its name from the genus *Arbutus* and is found in many related plants, including Pacific madrone (*Arbutus menziesii*), strawberry tree (*Arbutus unedo*), and all the species of *Arctostaphylos*.

This plant can also be used for other urinary tract issues that involve an inflamed urinary tract, such as urethritis, cystitis, poor bladder tone, and cloudy urine.

Uva ursi can be used topically for infections and as a douche for vaginal infections. Herbalist Sajah Popham even recommends using it internally for diarrhea because of its antibacterial and astringent qualities.

Making Medicine with Uva Ursi

Use the dried leaves for medicine. The most common method of preparation for uva ursi is as a hot infusion (tea). Some recommend it as a cold infusion, claiming that the antimicrobial constituents can be pulled out without extracting the astringent compounds that can hurt the stomach. For a cold infusion, crumble about a half cup of leaves in a 32-ounce mason jar, fill it with cold water, and put in the fridge to steep overnight. Strain it in the morning and drink 4 fluid ounces (½ cup) of this tea 3 to 4 times a day.

Tinctures are made with the dried leaves (see Tincture Ratio Chart). I don't typically use the tincture, because water reaches the kidneys and urinary system much more effectively, and alcohol is irritating to the bladder, which is counterproductive for the conditions this is used for.

Cautions

Uva ursi can be irritating to the stomach. Always combine it with a demulcent like marshmallow root, and limit internal use to short periods of no more than four days at a time. Stop taking immediately if you feel a burning hunger, heartburn, or other negative sensation in your stomach (which is around your solar plexus). It may be prudent to avoid use if you have a weak or irritated stomach already. Uva ursi is not for use during pregnancy.

Urinary tract infections can turn into kidney infections and cause death if not treated properly. Keep this in mind while using herbs to treat them. I have a personal 24-hour rule, which dictates that if the symptoms worsen within 24 hours of herbal treatment, I will go to the doctor or urgent care for medical help. Herbs are most effective at treating the early stages of an infection, when it is still mild. If a urinary tract infection progresses to the point that you have blood in your urine and flank pain, then it is already time to seek medical help.

Violet

Viola glabella, V. sempervirens
Violaceae (violet family)

There are violet species in temperate places throughout the world. They are all edible and share similar medicinal uses. All parts of the violet plant have been used for medicine. They have a rich and well-documented history of use in various cultures—including the Indigenous cultures of North America, Europe, and China—and are mentioned in the very first texts on plant medicine.

We have twenty-four wild species of violet in Washington State alone, most of which are native and many of which are fairly rare. Please avoid the rare species and harvest only where abundant! You can also help reduce pressure on the wild populations by planting violets in your garden. Butterflies enjoy them immensely.

Violets bloom so early in the year that their pollination can get interrupted by inclement weather. Because of this, they've adapted a backup option for producing seeds. Violets have a second set of blossoms in the fall that are underground and self-fertile, meaning those flowers don't require cross-pollination. Though the seeds from these flowers will not offer new genetic material, they still give the plant a chance to produce a new generation. Plants that do this are called cleistogamous.

LEFT A patch of stream violet (*V. glabella*) **RIGHT** A patch of evergreen violet (*V. sempervirens*) on the forest floor (Photo by Ben Legler)

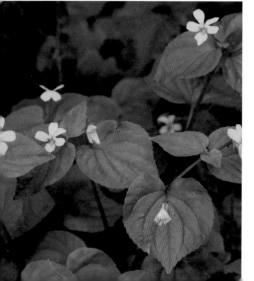 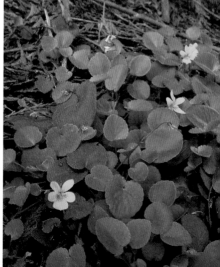

Stream violet *Viola glabella*	**Evergreen violet** *Viola sempervirens*
Flower 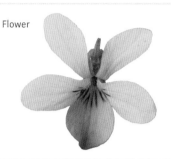	Flower (Photo by Ben Legler) 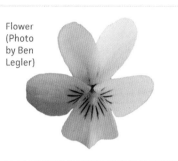
Leaf 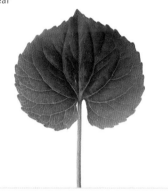	Leaf 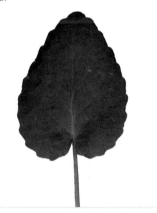

Whole plant

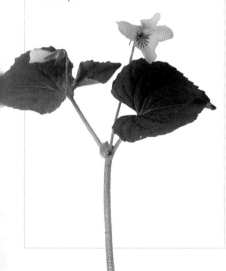

Look-Alike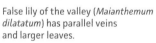

False lily of the valley (*Maianthemum dilatatum*) has parallel veins and larger leaves.

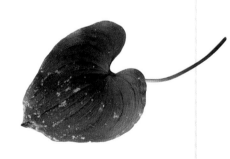

Harvesting Violet

Because violet is a bit more elusive than some of the other plants in this book, we need to be attentive to our impact on it. I harvest only when I find an abundant patch (which I define as more than 4 square feet), and I take only a leaf or two from each plant to ensure their success. There are a lot of rare violet species in our bioregion—like early blue violet (*Viola adunca*). Please enjoy those rarer species without harvesting.

Harvest the leaves in early spring, when they are the most tender; this is also the time when the flowers are in bloom. At sea level, they can sometimes even be found blooming in January and February if we have slightly warm weather. Farther up in the mountains, they will be the first to bloom when the snow recedes or the freezes begin to let up.

Stream violet (*Viola glabella*) is my favorite species to harvest in our region and is fairly abundant. As the name suggests, it grows along streams and in wet areas. I have found it in open areas at many elevations, sometimes growing in a ditch along a forest service road, sometimes in a wet and open meadow, and sometimes in a bigleaf maple grove among the bleeding hearts.

You can also harvest leaves from evergreen violet (*Viola sempervirens*), which is fairly abundant in our forests, but the

LEFT Harvesting the leaves and flowers of stream violet in very early spring **RIGHT** Heart-shaped leaves and palmate venation set violet leaves apart from look-alikes.

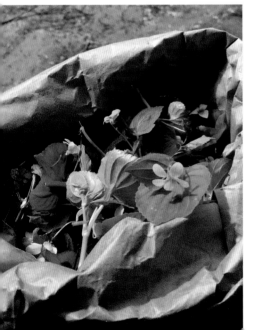
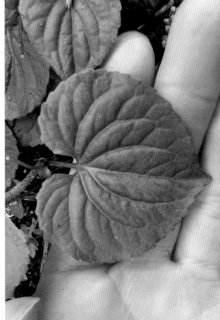

leaves are rather fibrous and higher in salicylic acid than other species. When you chew an evergreen violet leaf, eventually you will get a subtle hint of wintergreen flavor, which comes from the salicylic acid.

Consider growing sweet violet (*Viola odorata*) in your garden to supplement your wild harvests. Sweet violet is a European variety, and the flowers are famously delicious and sweet smelling. It is a perennial ground cover that loves moist places.

Medicinal Uses of Violet

Violet soothes inflammation, moistens tissues, reduces swelling, dissolves benign cysts and fatty deposits, and reduces lymphatic congestion. The leaf is used most often as it is the most abundant. I have used violet leaf mostly in tea formulas for reflux and gastrointestinal irritation.

One of the most common uses for violet leaf nowadays is for eczema. It is taken as a tea internally and used as a cream externally. Because it is cool and moist in nature, it is most useful for eczema with redness, dryness, and itching.

Violet is also a gentle lymphatic tonic and can be used with cleavers and red clover in a lymphatic cleansing tea (see Lymphatic Clearing Tea). This combination of herbs might be helpful if you have chronic swollen lymph nodes or are prone to cyst-like growths.

Interestingly, the roots and seeds have a history of use to induce vomiting, so avoid those unless that is desired.

The leaves and flowers of all violet species are edible and can be eaten raw in salads. The medicinal actions can be accessed in this way also!

Making Medicine with Violet

A tea made from the fresh or dried leaves is the main preparation when using violet for therapeutic purposes. To make an infusion with the fresh leaves, put a few handfuls of the leaves in a 32-ounce mason jar. Pour boiling water over the top, cover, and let sit overnight. In the morning, strain it and put it in the fridge. Drink the infusion cold throughout the day, and make a fresh batch daily. This does indeed take a lot of fresh leaves,

LYMPHATIC CLEARING TEA   *Makes 1.5 ounces loose-leaf tea*

This tea helps mobilize the lymphatic system, helping to rid you of toxins that accumulate there. A stagnant lymph system can cause skin issues. The tea takes equal parts violet leaf, cleavers, and red clover, so feel free to scale this recipe up or down.

Dosage: Use 1 to 2 tablespoons per cup of boiling water. Infuse for 10 minutes, covered. Strain and drink warm. Drink 1 cup daily, with honey if desired.

½ ounce dried violet leaf
½ ounce dried cleavers
½ ounce dried red clover

Combine all ingredients in a medium bowl. Transfer to a jar and store for up to 1 year.

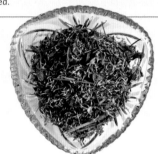

which is why making it with dried leaves is a bit more practical, though not as potent according to most sources.

I make an alcohol intermediary oil with leaves I have dried. Though it is more traditional to use slightly wilted fresh leaves and soak them in oil, the dried leaves make a more shelf-stable product and are easier to work with in this preparation than fresh leaves. It's also common to infuse the flowers in oil, though I rarely acquire enough flowers to do that.

A poultice of the fresh leaf can be used on swollen lymph nodes, which involves mashing up the leaves and making a paste that you apply to the area and cover with a cloth.

The flowers are also used, but it is incredibly painstaking to find enough to harvest. Many sources that discuss violet are specifically talking about sweet violet. There are a lot of preparations made with the scented and delicious flowers of sweet violet that may not translate to our native violet species, whose flowers don't have a strong taste or smell.

Cautions

Violet leaves contain salicylates, so avoid using them internally if there is a salicylate sensitivity.

Wild Carrot

Daucus carota
Apiaceae (carrot family)

Wild carrot is also known as Queen Anne's lace, a name that comes from a peculiar, single red flower in the very center of the inflorescence among many tiny white flowers (see photos). In a story that originated in the British Isles, the name is said to represent a drop of red blood that fell from Queen Anne's finger when she was making lace.

Wild carrot (*Daucus carota*) is actually the same species that our table carrot originates from—the root even smells like a carrot. Carrots were originally domesticated from wild carrot in central Asia, then also domesticated separately in Iran. Wild carrot is still a thriving weed in many parts of the world! It loves roadsides, paths, and grassy fields. You can eat the root of the wild carrot, though it is fibrous, aromatic, and small.

You can easily introduce wild carrot into your garden by collecting its seed in the fall. The seed should be brown and ready to just fall off the plant. Right after harvesting the seeds, sprinkle them in an area where you'd like wild carrot to grow. You can also plant the seeds in flats in the spring and then transplant the starts. There are garden varieties of Queen Anne's lace that are nice too. As long as the seeds smell strongly, they will bring you good medicine.

LEFT Identify wild carrot by the red blossom surrounded by tiny white flowers. **RIGHT** A spider hanging out in a cup-shaped seed head, which is prime for harvest

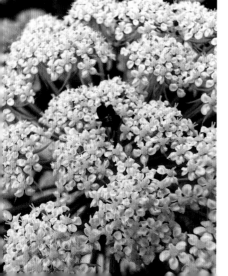 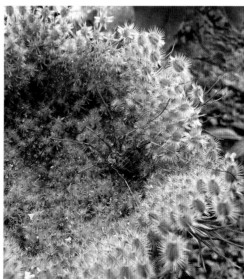

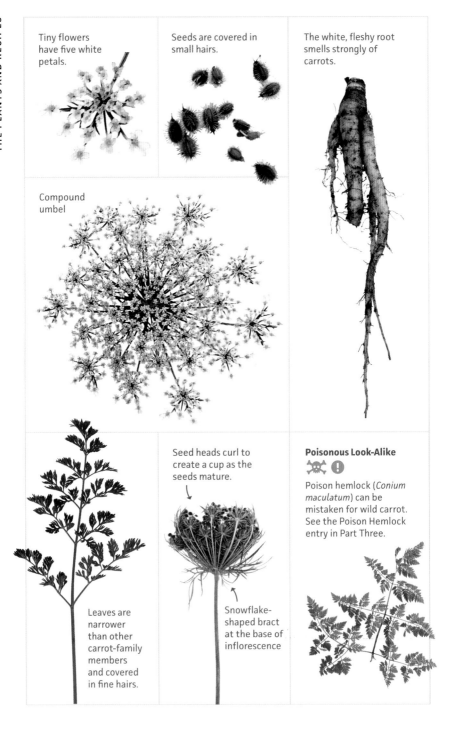

Tiny flowers have five white petals.

Seeds are covered in small hairs.

The white, fleshy root smells strongly of carrots.

Compound umbel

Leaves are narrower than other carrot-family members and covered in fine hairs.

Seed heads curl to create a cup as the seeds mature.

Snowflake-shaped bract at the base of inflorescence

Poisonous Look-Alike

Poison hemlock (*Conium maculatum*) can be mistaken for wild carrot. See the Poison Hemlock entry in Part Three.

Harvesting Wild Carrot

Wild carrot can be found mostly on the west side of the Cascades in grassy areas. It makes itself known especially in late summer.

Many people are paranoid about harvesting wild carrot because it is a member of the carrot family and grows in similar habitats to its poisonous cousin, poison hemlock (*Conium maculatum*). There are several distinct characteristics that make wild carrot easy to distinguish, but still be very careful when harvesting (see the Poison Hemlock entry in Part Three for more information and photos).

Wild carrot seeds begin ripening at the beginning of August and continue through September. I harvest the immature green seed heads, which smell very aromatic and sweet. Squeeze the seeds between your fingers to release the volatile oils and sniff to test. The seeds should be a bit plump, and the seed head should start to curl upward to create a cup. Snip the seed heads off into your bag with scissors or clippers. You can come back for more seeds later as the plants flower continuously.

Be aware that insects love to hang out in these seed heads. I once saw a ladybug and an earwig hanging out in one together! I shake the seed heads out a bit while harvesting so there are no big surprises crawling out in the car while I'm driving home. And yes, that is a lesson learned from experience.

Wild carrot seed is a very sustainable harvest, as it is a common weed. Just be careful not to harvest too close to busy roads or in a place that could have been sprayed or have soil contamination. Try looking in your local park or in a grassy field that hasn't been mowed. Carrot seeds from garden carrots can also be used, though they are less potent than the wild type.

You can harvest the flowers starting in late July, extending into early September. Pick flowers that have just opened and look fresh. Also watch for bugs in these, especially cute little white spiders that blend in with the white flowers.

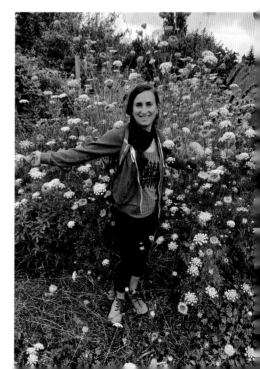

This patch of wild carrot was a lucky find!

Medicinal Uses of Wild Carrot

Wild carrot seed has been used for a long time as a female contraceptive, as mentioned by Dioscorides in his famous book *De materia medica* more than two thousand years ago.

In modern times, this plant continues to be used by many female-bodied people as a contraceptive, and results are mixed. I know multiple people who have conceived while taking wild carrot preventatively, so I don't recommend it. In fact, wild carrot seed may actually work to aid fertility in the long run, and has been used for that historically. If you are interested in using wild carrot seed as a contraceptive, research not only dosage and frequency but also its mechanism of action, which

WILD CARROT HYDROSOL
Makes about 8 ounces

A hydrosol is a distilled aromatic liquid made with plants. You can make your own still at home, which does not yield as much as a large copper still would, but it works quite well if you can find the right pot. Make sure you have plenty of ice on hand for this preparation; you will also need a gallon-size resealable bag. Hydrosols can be made from any plant, though aromatic plants are especially good. Apply a few sprays of hydrosol underneath a face oil or serum to add extra moisture, use it as the liquid component in creams, or use it as a room spray. This hydrosol is best for external use only.

8 cups fresh wild carrot seed heads
4 to 6 cups water, plus 1 to 2 tablespoons
  for the rye paste
4 tablespoons rye flour

Choose a deep pot with a convex lid that can be fitted upside down. The shape is important, because the condensed steam must be able to drip downward at a central point.

Put a small bowl upside down in the bottom of the pot, and then another small bowl right side up on top of it. Nestle the carrot seed heads around this central tower (see photo).

Add the water to the pot, making sure that the water does not go above the bottom bowl, which would cause the top bowl to float off.

Put the lid upside down on the top of the pot. The lid should not touch the bowls or the plant material.

In a small bowl, make a paste with the flour and water; start with 1 tablespoon of water and add a bit more as needed to make a smooth, sticky paste. Use your fingers to smear the paste around the rim of the pot, where the upside-down lid sits (see photo). This seals the lid and prevents precious steam from escaping.

are outside the scope of this book. When you are dealing with a high-stakes use like this, always draw from several sources.

Wild carrot seed is also an emmenagogue (it brings on menstruation), diuretic, gastroprotective, nephroprotective (protects the kidneys), and aphrodisiac. It has many, many other actions.

Wild carrot has a history of use in herbal traditions across Eurasia, including Ayurveda, traditional Persian medicine, and in many European traditions. One universal use for it is removing obstructions in the body, especially in the liver. This use makes sense because aromatic herbs tend to be moving and opening in nature. Also along those lines, it is used as a stomach tonic to address flatulence and slow digestion. Most traditions

Set the pot over medium heat. As soon as it starts to get hot, fill a resealable gallon bag with ice, seal, and set the bag on top of the inverted lid. Once the water starts to boil and you hear the bubbles, reduce the heat to low to simmer gently. Simmer for 20 minutes, replacing the ice as soon as most of it has melted. To replace ice, pour out the water from the previous batch and refill the same bag with fresh ice. For me, it takes two to three batches of ice. During this time, the hydrosol will collect in the center bowl as it steams up and is condensed on the top by the cold ice.

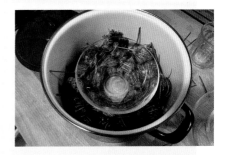

Do not open the lid to check until you are done, as it will interrupt the operation and allow precious steam to escape. Unfortunately there is not a good way to check whether your setup is working, so it's a bit of a blind faith project. When the time is up, turn off the heat and let cool for a few minutes. Once it's cool enough to handle, break the seal using a butter knife and remove the lid from the top, and hopefully there will be aromatic liquid in the bowl!

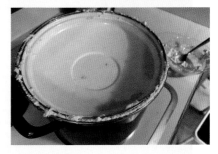

Transfer the hydrosol to an 8-ounce bottle. The hydrosol will keep for 1 to 3 years and is best kept in the fridge.

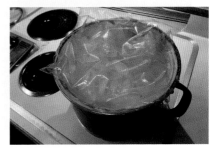

also mention its use for the bladder and kidneys—especially for stones. Most of these uses have fallen out of favor in modern times.

Nowadays, essential oil made from wild carrot seed is the most widely known and available form of wild carrot. It is used in wrinkle creams, sunscreens, and acne formulas. It is also used in a lot of skincare products for anti-aging. It is apparently firming, antioxidant, clearing, and anti-inflammatory.

Making Medicine with Wild Carrot

The immature green seed is the main part of this plant used for medicine. They should smell sweet and spicy when crushed. I make a tincture of these green seeds, blending them with the alcohol to get a good extraction (see Tincture Ratio Chart). Remove as much stem as you can before tincturing.

Some people also grind the seed or chew it fresh, which I have seen recommended specifically when using it as a contraceptive (but see Medicinal Uses of Wild Carrot for more on this use).

Wild carrot seed is also used extensively in skin care products. I make a hydrosol to spray on my face before using a face oil (see Wild Carrot Hydrosol). You can also make a traditional infused oil or an alcohol intermediary oil. You could even add some wild carrot essential oil to strengthen it—for this, add 5 to 10 drops per fluid ounce of oil.

The flowers can be dried for tea. They aren't used much for medicine, but they produce a really nice, complex floral tea that has notes of Earl Grey.

Cautions

Wild carrot seed is not safe to use during pregnancy or breastfeeding. It should also be avoided in cases of kidney failure and in folks with interstitial cystitis, as it can irritate the kidney and the bladder's lining. It is stimulating and a bit irritating and thus should be avoided by those with a hot constitution, who are already prone to being stimulated and irritated.

Willow

Salix spp.
Salicaceae (willow family)

Many willows grow wild in our bioregion, yet very few taste good enough to use for medicine. My advice for you: Find a willow tree you like the taste of and continue to visit it. Harvest from other willows for topical use or to make baskets and cordage.

With some exceptions, these lovely trees generally grow near water. Willows are very important to our wetland ecosystems as they help filter the water and prevent flooding.

Harvesting Willow

I harvest willow bark in April, when the bark is wet and slips easily off the branch. It also tastes best at this stage of growth. For the best medicine, select a branch thicker than your thumb and remove at a node with clippers or a saw. Peel the bark off the branch with fingers or a pocketknife. Peeling should be done as soon as possible after harvesting, because it will be more difficult to peel as it dries. You can make medicine with the fresh bark, or dry it and store it for later use.

Willow is easily propagated due to its large amount of growth hormones. You can stick a branch in the ground and it will grow into a new tree! When you cut a branch off a willow tree, it will usually send out numerous shoots in its place. Because of this

LEFT Willow seeds forming. The small capsules of each catkin will open and release fuzz when the seeds are ready. **RIGHT** In the spring, the bark will often come off easily. This is also when you harvest for basketmaking.

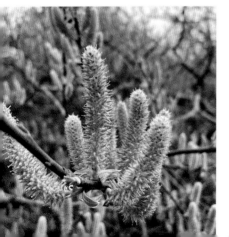
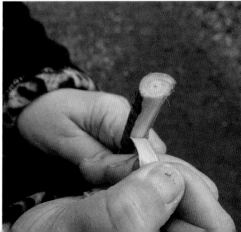

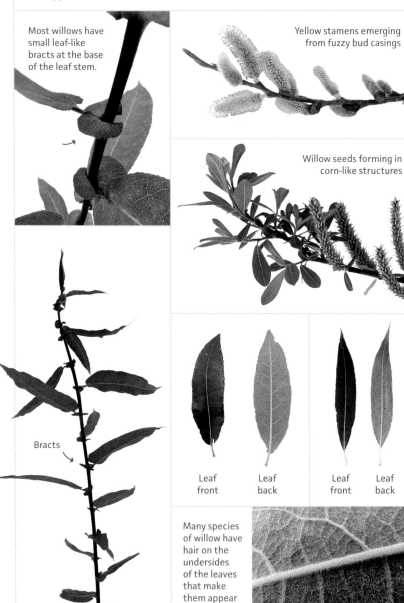

Various willow species
Salix spp.

Most willows have small leaf-like bracts at the base of the leaf stem.

Yellow stamens emerging from fuzzy bud casings

Willow seeds forming in corn-like structures

Bracts

Leaf front

Leaf back

Leaf front

Leaf back

Many species of willow have hair on the undersides of the leaves that make them appear silver.

vigorous response to cutting, this is a very sustainable plant to harvest.

The long and straight first-year branches of willow are used in weaving because of their flexibility and strength. A pruning technique called coppicing is used to encourage first-year suckers for weaving. Coppicing involves cutting all the branches to the ground in the winter. Throughout the year, hundreds of new thin branches grow up from the stump and are all cut again the next winter. A willow tree can survive this process for up to sixty years!

Medicinal Uses of Willow

Willow bark is famously the original source of aspirin, which is now made in a lab. Like aspirin, willow bark is used for pain caused by inflammation, which includes headaches, joint pain, menstrual cramps, tooth pain, and more, but it is far gentler on the stomach than aspirin due to the presence of protective compounds.

Dosage is very important when using willow bark for pain. Its effects aren't as long lasting as over-the-counter painkillers like ibuprofen, so you need to dose it a bit more frequently. Each person will need to find their sweet spot, but I dose 1 dropperful of the tincture every hour. I typically also take a larger initial dose of 2 dropperfuls. Keep in mind that if your tincture is weaker (if it's not standardized), then you may need to take more in a dose for the same effect.

LEFT Harvesting willow bark in February. Choose branches thicker than your thumb.
RIGHT Peeling willow bark on a riverbank. You will always find willow near water.

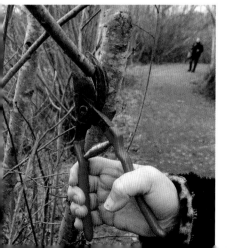
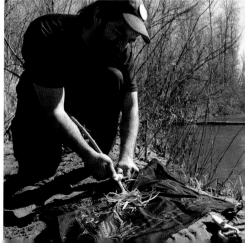

For menstrual cramps, I combine willow bark tincture with cramp bark tincture (equal parts of each). For migraines, I combine willow bark with the tinctures of lavender and feverfew.

Willow bark can also be used topically for pain and inflammation in many different ways. You can make a tea and rinse your mouth with it for inflamed gums after dental procedures. To prevent infection as well, add Oregon grape bark to the mouth rinse. A willow bark foot bath is great for painful feet from walking or injury. A willow infused oil could be used to treat painful joints, though that's not the best way to extract the active constituents of willow bark. Willow bark is best extracted in water, alcohol, or vinegar.

Making Medicine with Willow

A tincture of spring willow bark is the most common preparation of this plant (see Tincture of Dried Willow Bark). Many of our local willow species may have too strong a taste for internal use. I have found a few willow trees in my area that have bark tolerable enough to be made into a tincture. Taste some of your local species and see what you think.

TINCTURE OF DRIED WILLOW BARK   *Makes about 10 ounces*

Willow bark tincture is a mainstay of my herbal first aid kit. It is the first tincture I reach for when I have a headache or a musculoskeletal injury with swelling. If you are working with longer pieces, break them up.

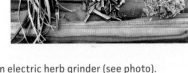

Dosage: Take 30 to 60 drops every 1 to 2 hours while the pain persists.

2.5 ounces dried willow bark, broken up into small pieces
12.5 fluid ounces 100-proof alcohol (50 percent), such as vodka

Grind the bark pieces into shreds using an electric herb grinder (see photo).

Put the shredded bark in a clean 16-ounce jar with the alcohol, secure the lid, and shake well.

Label well and let sit in a cool, dark place for 4 weeks, shaking occasionally, and then strain with a fine-mesh strainer.

Store in a 16-ounce jar for up to 5 years.

WILLOW BARK INFUSED WITCH HAZEL   *Makes about 11 ounces*

Put this infused witch hazel in a spray bottle and apply to sunburns and after any type of hair removal that can irritate hair follicles and leave redness. It is soothing, astringent, and anti-inflammatory. You can follow with plantain infused oil (make your own using the technique described in the Bleeding Heart Alcohol Intermediary Oil recipe).
This recipe is designed to use one 12-ounce bottle of store-bought witch hazel—a liquid astringent used for first aid and skin care.

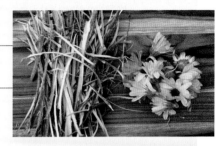

Dosage: Spray the affected area several times a day as needed.

1½ cups packed fresh willow bark
½ cup fresh or dried calendula flowers
12 fluid ounces witch hazel

Loosely pack the bark and flowers into a clean 16-ounce jar.
　Pour the witch hazel over the herbs to cover.
　Let sit in a cool, dark place for 1 month, then strain out the plant material using cheesecloth.
　Store in a plastic, glass, or metal spray bottle for up to 1 year.

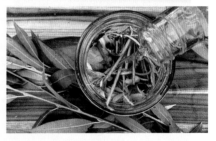

　The other preparation that I really love is Willow Bark Infused Witch Hazel (see recipe). I have also made willow bark hydrosol, which is much like witch hazel in its action. Witch hazel is actually just a hydrosol of the witch hazel tree, which is favored for its astringency. Willow bark is also very astringent and has the added benefit of being anti-inflammatory. It would make a great toner for acne-prone or inflamed skin. See the Wild Carrot Hydrosol recipe for instructions on preparing a hydrosol.

Cautions

Like aspirin, willow bark thins the blood, so do not take it with any blood-thinning medications.

Yarrow

Achillea millefolium
Asteraceae (sunflower family)

Yarrow is found in every single corner of the US and many more places around the world. It is very versatile in habitat, able to grow in subalpine meadows, deserts, suburban median strips, and coastal cliffs, to name a few. Yarrow has a uniquely large genetic variance for one species. Some yarrow is fuzzy and small, some is large, some is more aromatic, and some is short.

There is evidence to suggest yarrow has been used medicinally by humans as far back as 60,000 years ago, with many of the historical uses matching up across cultures and continents. The genus, *Achillea*, is named after the Greek Achilles, who used yarrow ointments for his soldiers.

Harvesting Yarrow

The flowering tops are the part of yarrow used most often for medicine. Harvest the freshly opening flower heads when it has just begun to bloom. June is typically the best month to harvest, but you can find fresh blooms from May to September. The aromatic content of older flower heads will not be as good. Yarrow that grows in drier parts of our bioregion (like in a sagebrush

LEFT Yarrow growing in a grassy meadow along with hairy cat's ear **RIGHT** A close-up of the compound flowers of yarrow. Flowers sometimes have a pink tinge.

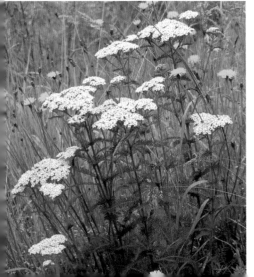
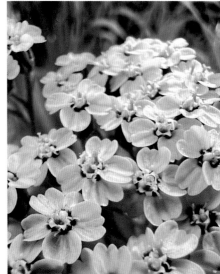

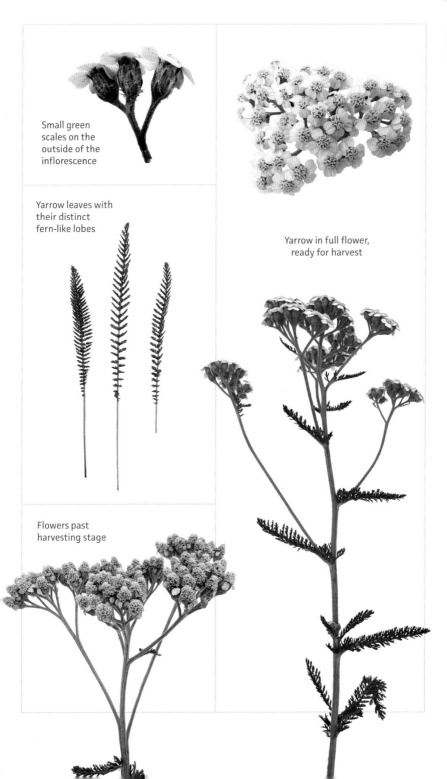

Small green scales on the outside of the inflorescence

Yarrow leaves with their distinct fern-like lobes

Yarrow in full flower, ready for harvest

Flowers past harvesting stage

steppe on the east side of the Cascades) will be the most aromatic. In general, plants in drier climates tend to produce more aromatics.

The leaves of yarrow can also be harvested and are most typically used fresh to stop bleeding. They can be harvested at any time. I always have yarrow growing in my garden so I can have it on hand. This is definitely a great plant to introduce to your garden, as it is incredibly popular among pollinators, makes a great cut flower, and does not need much water, if any. To plant in your garden, dig up a few seedlings from the wild and plant directly into the soil. Yarrow will spread and come back year after year.

Yarrow is abundant in many places in our area. Harvest where it is plentiful, and don't take all the flowers. I avoid harvesting from populations in more sensitive habitats, such as subalpine zones.

Medicinal Uses of Yarrow

Fresh yarrow leaf can be used topically as a poultice to stop or slow bleeding. This action is called styptic. Chew or crush a bit of the leaf and stick it up a nostril to stop a nosebleed. I have successfully used a yarrow leaf poultice to stop the bleeding on cuts from sharp knives, which are deep and bleed freely.

Used internally, yarrow can increase circulation and relieve blood stagnation. The blood-moving action is often employed in formulas, along with other blood-movers such as angelica and mugwort, to resolve blood stagnation in the uterus. It is also used as an emmenagogue, which stimulates menstruation.

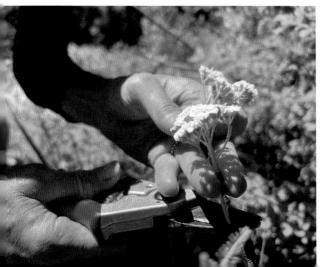

Harvesting the freshly opened flowering tops of yarrow in a large, open meadow

Yarrow is also a diaphoretic, which means it opens your pores and makes you sweat. It is used to break fevers, usually as a hot tea to increase the sweating action. If you are going to use it for a fever, be sure to use it at the onset of the fever and not four days in—a bit of wisdom borrowed from Chinese medicine (see Classic Cold and Flu Tea Blend recipe).

Yarrow is also aromatic and bitter, which means it is an herb for phlegmy coughs. For this, you can combine it with other gentle cough herbs like mullein, thyme, elderflower, and goldenrod. There are also references to yarrow being used for stomach complaints historically, though herbalists don't often use it for that nowadays.

CLASSIC COLD AND FLU TEA BLEND   *Makes 1.5 ounces*

Drink this tea hot with honey. It should make you sweat, so feel free to bundle up in bed and sweat it out. I pull the yarrow flowers off the stems before blending them into teas.

Dosage: Use 1 tablespoon per cup. Infuse for 10 minutes, covered. Drink 2 to 3 cups a day at the first sign of a cold or flu.

0.6 ounce dried elderflower
0.5 ounce dried peppermint leaf
0.4 ounce dried yarrow flowering tops

Combine all ingredients in a large bowl and mix well.

Transfer to a clean 16-ounce jar and store for up to 2 years.

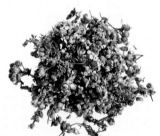

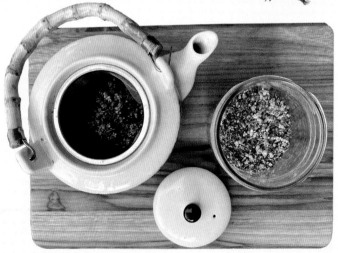

THE PLANTS AND RECIPES

Making Medicine with Yarrow

The most useful preparation of yarrow is a hot infusion, though it does not taste great. I combine it with other herbs in a formula and add honey to the hot tea. Remember to cover the tea while it steeps to keep the volatile oils intact.

To make a fresh leaf poultice to stop or slow bleeding, harvest a few leaves, chew them or otherwise break them down into a paste, and apply to the wound. Leave on for fifteen minutes or so and clean the area well afterward. Some people also make a fine powder of dried yarrow flowers, which they put in a small tin in their herbal first aid kit. The idea is to sprinkle the powder onto a cut to stop the bleeding.

You can make a tincture of the fresh or dry flowering tops (see Tincture Ratio Chart). The tincture will not help with bleeding cuts, though, as alcohol reverses any styptic actions the yarrow might have. The tincture is best for internal use, primarily in cough formulas, cold and flu formulas, and blood stagnation formulas.

A set of fifty dried, trimmed yarrow stalks are used in the process of reading the *I-Ching*, an ancient Chinese divination method. The stalks are used to produce random numbers by dividing, counting, and then dividing again. Check it out if you're feeling adventurous!

Cautions

Do not use yarrow during pregnancy. It also has some potential drug interactions, so do your research before using it internally if you are on any medications.

Yellow Dock

Rumex crispus
Polygonaceae (buckwheat family)

Yellow dock, also known as curly dock, was introduced to our continent from Europe. It grows all over the US and is considered a noxious weed in many states. Yellow dock is a perennial, coming back from the same root stalk year after year. The roots of older plants will have developed more medicinal compounds and are often sought after for this reason.

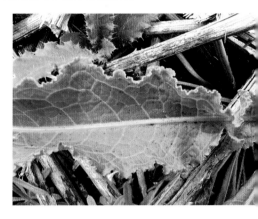

This plant can be found in both wet and dry areas of the bioregion, and in both wild areas and heavily developed areas. I find it growing most frequently in muddy areas of seasonal wetness, like ditches and low spots in fields. Its habitat (mud) reflects its use as a cleaner of a boggy large intestine.

The characteristic curly leaf edges and red spots along the central vein

Broadleaf dock (*Rumex obtusifolius*) looks quite similar but does not have the same medicinal actions. There are also other species of dock that might look similar but are much more rare. The yellow root, curled leaf edges, and narrower leaf shape are a good way to distinguish yellow dock from broadleaf dock (see photos).

LEFT The yellow roots for which yellow dock is named. Darker yellow roots are best.
RIGHT Harvesting yellow dock root in a local community garden

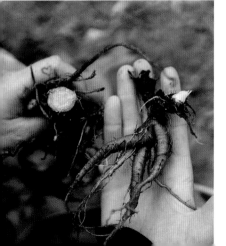

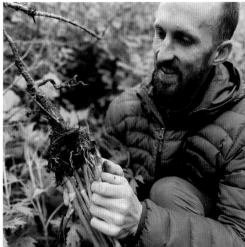

254

THE PLANTS AND RECIPES

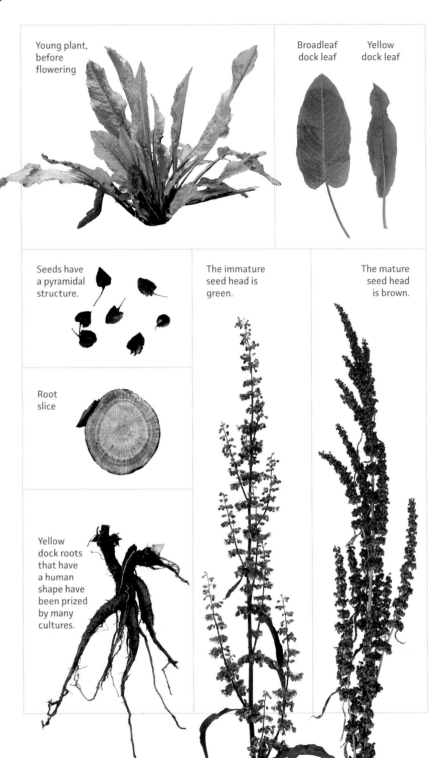

Young plant, before flowering

Broadleaf dock leaf

Yellow dock leaf

Seeds have a pyramidal structure.

The immature seed head is green.

The mature seed head is brown.

Root slice

Yellow dock roots that have a human shape have been prized by many cultures.

Harvesting Yellow Dock

Harvest yellow dock roots in spring when the flower stalk has not yet emerged and the plant is still just a cluster of leaves coming out of the root crown. When the plant is flowering or in seed, the root has significantly less vitality and thus less medicine in it. You may be able to harvest in the fall as well, but I have trouble finding plants that haven't gone to seed by then.

Yellow dock root is a very sustainable harvest due to its widespread, weedy habit, though please don't dig up every plant you see. If there are only a few plants in an area, follow the one-in-ten rule—for every ten plants you see, dig up one. To harvest the root, use a digging fork to loosen the soil to get as much of the taproot as possible. Plants with a wider base are going to have a wider root. The darker yellow the root is, the better the medicine will be. Hose off the roots when you get home and then scrub them with a brush.

The leaves of both yellow dock and broadleaf dock are best harvested for eating when very young and tender, usually in March through May (but see Cautions). The seeds mature in August and are still available through September. Wait until the seeds turn brown and begin to dry out to harvest, but don't wait until they are moldy and falling off the stalk.

You can introduce yellow dock into your garden by harvesting mature seeds and broadcasting them. In my area, broadleaf

Washing yellow dock root with a hose to get most of the dirt off before bringing it home

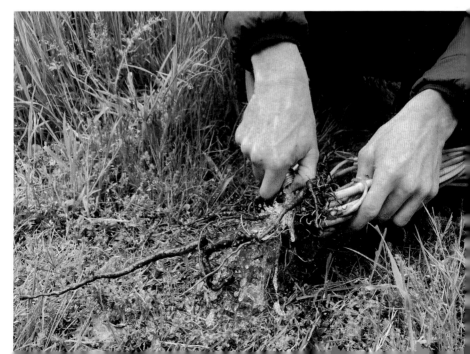

dock is unfortunately much more abundant, and it can sometimes be hard to come across a good yellow dock patch. I tend the patches that I find and make sure they stick around.

Medicinal Uses of Yellow Dock

Yellow dock root is bitter, astringent, and cooling, acting on the liver, large intestine, and, to some extent, the lungs. There are a lot of remedies that work on a congested liver, but not many that specialize in a sluggish large intestine, so that is where this plant shines.

FRESH TINCTURE OF YELLOW DOCK ROOT
Makes 8 to 10 ounces

Yellow dock tincture can be made with fresh or dried root, but when I harvest my own I make it fresh. Chop the yellow dock root as finely as possible with a knife. Do your best with the fibrous roots, using clippers if they are too woody for a knife.

This is a standardized tincture, meaning that a ratio is used to determine the ratio of alcohol to plant material. I also add 10 percent vegetable glycerin as this is one of the plants that can get gloppy at the bottom, and the glycerin helps those compounds stay in solution.

Dosage: Take 10 to 20 drops 2 to 3 times a day when symptoms are present.

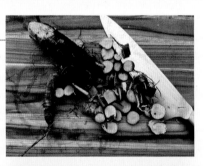

5 ounces fresh yellow dock root, finely chopped
5 fluid ounces 190-proof alcohol (95 percent), such as Everclear
4 fluid ounces water
1 fluid ounce vegetable glycerin

Put the chopped root into a clean 16-ounce jar, and pour the alcohol, water, and glycerin into the jar. Put the lid on and give it a good shake.

Label well, making sure to note the added glycerin.

Let sit in a cool, dark place, shaking occasionally, for 1 month. Then use cheesecloth to strain and return to the original jar.

Store in a cool, dark place for up to 5 years.

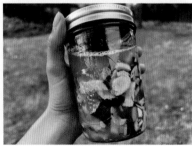

Use yellow dock root tincture for a sluggish and irritated large intestine, with loose but difficult-to-evacuate stool. Other indications for the use of yellow dock are bits of undigested food in the stool, food allergies, and slow transit time. Take 10 to 20 drops twice a day—in the morning before eating and in the evening before bed.

The root is a laxative, though its laxative compounds are far fewer than its cousin rhubarb root. The laxative effect comes from a group of compounds called anthraquinones that irritate the intestines and cause a bowel movement. Most sources say to use yellow dock in larger doses for constipation, though I would use rhubarb if it's available.

The yellow color of the root points toward its action on the liver and gallbladder. Specifically, it decongests the liver, which can be helpful in skin diseases, digestive disorders, and even chronic vaginal or bladder infections. It is a classic internal remedy for eczema especially, and will be best for weepy, red eczema outbreaks.

I once volunteered at the first aid tent at a gathering in Florida, and one of the other volunteers used yellow dock root tincture topically for fire-ant bites. We ended up mixing it with baking soda, another classic fire-ant remedy, to make a thick paste that we applied with success to several people who had bites all over their legs. Thankfully, we don't have fire ants in the Pacific Northwest, but I have heard others recommend the root for all insect bites.

The use of yellow dock in iron supplements is, apparently, not because it contains iron. Rather, it helps with the assimilation of iron and helps release iron stored in the liver.

Making Medicine with Yellow Dock

Most often, I make a tincture of the root (see Tincture Ratio Chart). You can use either the fresh or dried root, but I use it fresh as it has a stronger flavor (see Fresh Tincture of Yellow Dock Root). This tincture is a bit different because you add 10 percent glycerin to the menstruum. The glycerin stabilizes the tannins and prevents them from becoming a gooey mass at the bottom.

Dried yellow dock root can be used to make a tea. It is not tasty, but the tea can be used topically as a wash for boils and skin infections. Yellow dock is also a common ingredient in syrups for anemia, along with other iron-rich herbs like nettle.

Yellow dock leaves are edible, though they contain oxalic acid, which can be harmful to the kidneys in large amounts. Oxalic acid is found in many other edible plants, such as spinach, miner's lettuce, sheep sorrel, wood sorrel, and lambsquarters. Oxalic acid can be removed by boiling the plant in water and discarding the water. Plants like this are often harvested along with other plants and boiled together. This method of eating smaller amounts mixed in with other species is a great way to avoid overeating slightly toxic plants.

You can also eat the seeds ground into a flour, something that wilderness survivalists and daring wild foodies love to try. Before globalized food trade, it was common to supplement wheat flour with foraged items, like yellow dock seed meal, to extend them and add nutrition. I have seen people make yellow dock seed crackers mixed with other seeds, nuts, and flours.

Cautions

Yellow dock leaf contains oxalates that can damage the kidneys in large doses. Yellow dock root can be very drying and should be used with caution for dry or constipated individuals. Also, because it contains anthraquinones, taking too much could cause intestinal cramping and diarrhea.

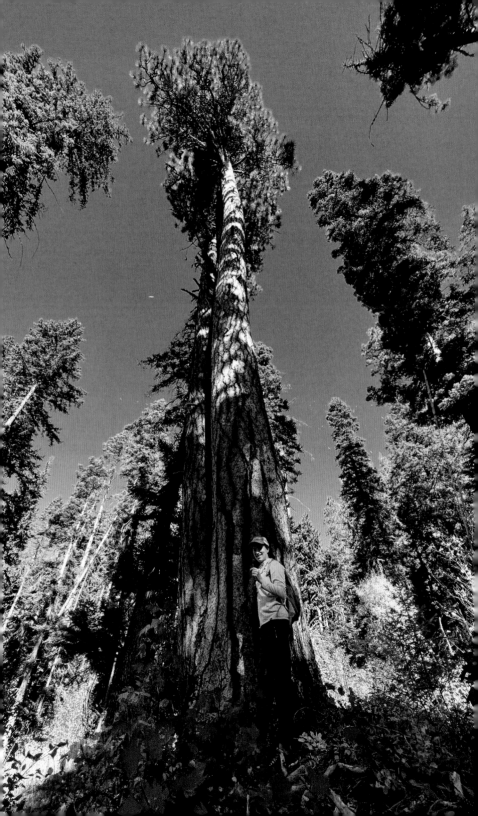

False hellebore about to bloom in an open field at a summer camp near Cle Elum, Washington

Part Three

Poisonous and Toxic Plants

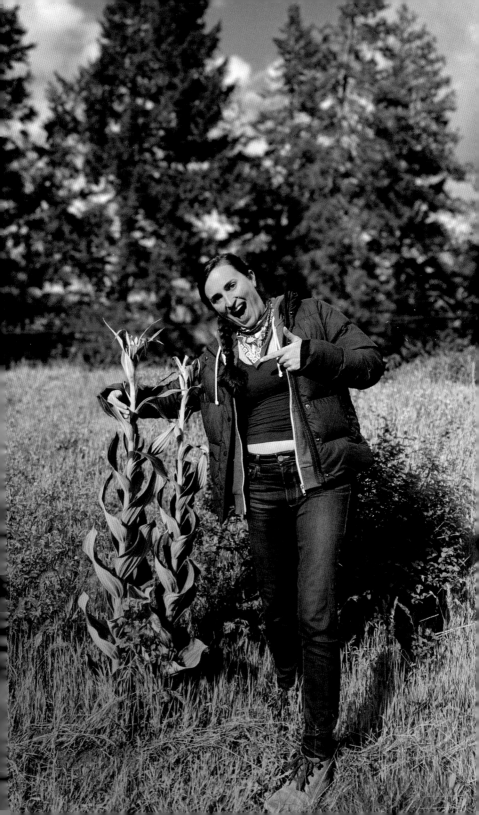

The plant entries in the following pages describe and depict some common toxic and poisonous plants in our bioregion to help you identify them. Supplement the information in this book with the Burke Herbarium Image Collection (see Resources), as well as digital pamphlets about poisonous and toxic plants from your state's Department of Transportation and Department of Agriculture. And remember my number-one rule for foraging: don't put it in your mouth until you are 100 percent certain of what it is.

Poisonous Plants

Learning to identify poisonous plants is just as important as learning to identify the plants you are out to forage. Poisonous plants are those that may be fatal if ingested. This section lists some of the most common poisonous plants in our area, but the list is in no way exhaustive, and only a handful of these are profiled in this section. Take extra care not to harvest these plants by accident to prevent getting even a single leaf or piece of root in your bag.

The seven most poisonous plants in the Pacific Northwest are

- Columbian monkshood (*Aconitum columbianum*)
- death camas (*Zigadenus venenosus*)
- false hellebore (*Veratrum* spp.)
- foxglove (*Digitalis purpurea*)
- larkspur (*Delphinium* spp.)
- poison hemlock (*Conium maculatum*)
- water hemlock (*Cicuta* spp.)

Consuming even just a little bit of these plants could be fatal. The seeds and roots are often the most poisonous parts of the plant. If you suspect you have consumed some, grab a sample, call poison control, and get yourself to the emergency room immediately. There are plenty of documented cases of poisoning that would have been fatal if not for the emergency interventions used in hospitals. These interventions are made easier when the doctors know what species was consumed, as the treatment may be different for each.

Toxic Plants

Toxic plants are not the same as poisonous. Though toxic plants may be fatal in large doses, they are more typically harmful in a nonfatal way. Arnica, for example, causes extreme gastrointestinal distress if taken internally. Many medicinal plants are toxic, in fact, and it is actually their toxins that make them so medicinally useful. There is a Greek adage that says, "The difference between a medicine and a poison is the dose."

Some examples of common toxic plants that grow in the Pacific Northwest are

- arnica (*Arnica* spp.)
- bittersweet nightshade (*Solanum dulcamara*)
- buttercup (*Ranunculus* spp.)
- chokecherry (*Prunus virginiana*)
- lupine (*Lupinus* spp.)
- poison oak (*Toxicodendron* spp.)

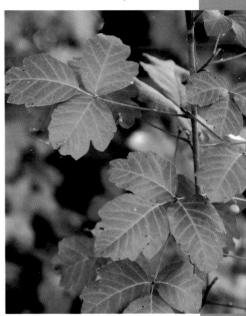

Pacific poison oak (*Toxicodendron diversilobium*) is a local toxic plant.

Some toxic plants, like poison oak, can cause an adverse reaction on the skin just by touching them. Some that you will find in the Pacific Northwest include

- devil's club (*Oplopanax horridus*)
- giant hogweed (*Heracleum mantegazzianum*)
- stinging nettle (*Urtica* spp.)

Hemiparasitic Plants

Some plants borrow nutrients from the plants around them. They are called hemiparasitic. Lousewort (*Pedicularis* spp.) is a good example of this. I haven't included any medicinal hemiparasitic plants in this book, but if you move into foraging these kinds of plants, they should absolutely not be harvested near poisonous or toxic species, as they may take up toxins from those plants and store them in their own tissues.

Bittersweet Nightshade ☠

Solanum dulcamara
Solanaceae (nightshade family)

Bittersweet nightshade is considered toxic, but not poisonous like the related plant deadly nightshade (*Atropa belladonna*), which does not grow wild in our bioregion. However, it still can cause nausea and even death if consumed in large doses. This is a red berry to avoid—look for the star-shaped stem attachment on the top of the berry. The leaves are irregularly lobed. This vining plant thrives in wetland environments, among cattail, red osier dogwood, and reed canary grass, for example.

Toxic symptoms could include nausea, vomiting, elevated heart rate, and potentially feelings of numbness or paralysis.

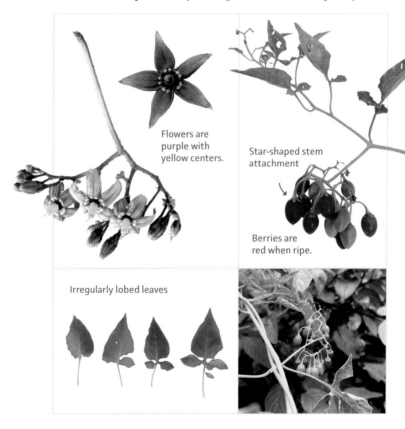

Flowers are purple with yellow centers.

Star-shaped stem attachment

Berries are red when ripe.

Irregularly lobed leaves

Columbian Monkshood ☠

Aconitum columbianum
Ranunculaceae (buttercup family)

This is a Pacific Northwest native species of the genus *Aconitum*, which is famously poisonous. It gets the name monkshood from its hooded flowers. It has also been known as wolfsbane and was thought to repel werewolves. The history of this plant is steeped in magical lore and, of course, death.

It is said that when you have been poisoned by monkshood, you will feel like ants are crawling all over your body. There may also be facial numbness, weakness in the limbs, cardiovascular symptoms, nausea, and vomiting. Like other plant poisons, this is a central nervous system sedative that can cause asphyxiation and death with even just a little bit consumed.

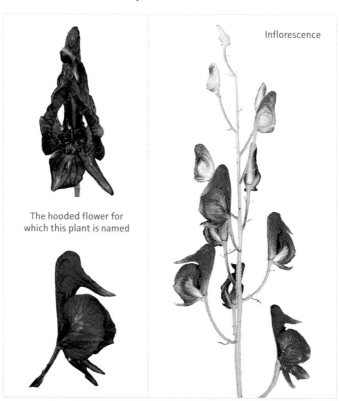

Inflorescence

The hooded flower for which this plant is named

False Hellebore ☠

Veratrum viride, V. californicum
Melianthiaceae (false hellebore family)

American false hellebore (*Veratrum viride*), pictured here, is a plant of moist meadows and open woodlands. It is most common at higher elevations but can occasionally be found as low as sea level. Its range is broad in Oregon, Washington, British Columbia, and into the southern parts of Alaska. As the name suggests, California false hellebore (*Veratrum californicum*), not pictured here, is found only occasionally in Washington and is more common in California, southern Oregon, and in the Sierras and Rockies.

This highly poisonous plant slows heart rate, interferes with normal electrical functions in the heart, and can cause a drop in blood pressure.

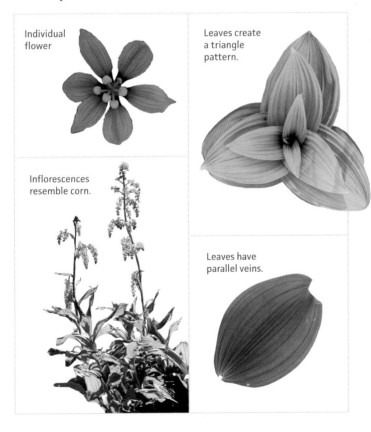

Individual flower

Leaves create a triangle pattern.

Inflorescences resemble corn.

Leaves have parallel veins.

Foxglove ☠

Digitalis purpurea
Scrophulariaceae (figwort family)

Strangely, though foxglove is highly poisonous, it is a popular cut flower and garden plant. You can often find entire hillsides in full bloom in June and July, which are absolutely beautiful—just give them space when harvesting nearby. Before flowering, foxglove looks a lot like mullein (*Verbascum* spp.), so take care when harvesting mullein that does not have flowers.

Foxglove is a cardiac depressant, causing slowed heartbeat and low blood pressure. Because of its marked effect on the heart, it is the original source of the pharmaceutical digoxin, a heart medication.

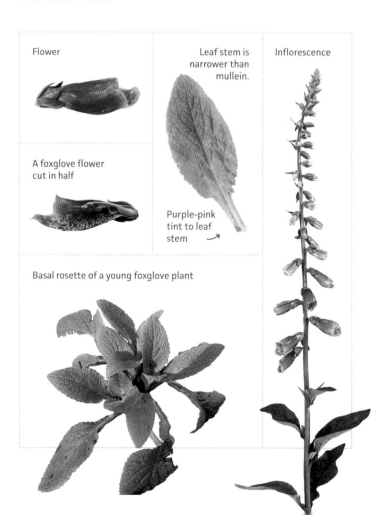

Flower

A foxglove flower cut in half

Leaf stem is narrower than mullein.

Purple-pink tint to leaf stem ↗

Inflorescence

Basal rosette of a young foxglove plant

Larkspur ☠

Delphinium spp.
Ranunculaceae (buttercup family)

In the Pacific Northwest, there are many species of the *Delphinium* genus, and all share the common name larkspur. Flowers range from white to deep purple. This is one of my favorite wildflowers because of the shocking purple color. It grows in patches, often in open meadows, and is more common in the drier parts of the region, east of the Cascades, and in our prairies.

Larkspur is sometimes confused with monkshood. To distinguish larkspur from monkshood, note the flower shape. Monkshood has a hooded flower (see the Columbian Monkshood entry in this section), whereas larkspur has a characteristic spur at the back of each flower.

This plant is fatal to humans when ingested, working similarly to its cousin, Monkshood (*Aconitum* spp.).

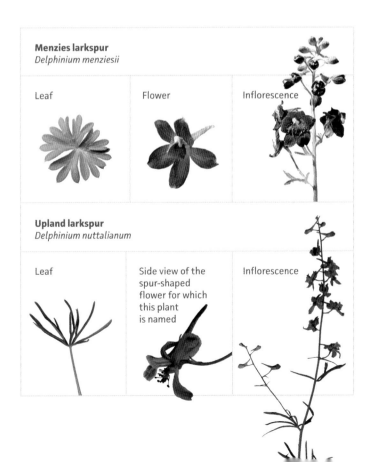

Menzies larkspur
Delphinium menziesii

Leaf | Flower | Inflorescence

Upland larkspur
Delphinium nuttalianum

Leaf | Side view of the spur-shaped flower for which this plant is named | Inflorescence

Poison Hemlock ☠

Conium maculatum
Apiaceae (carrot family)

Poison hemlock is perhaps the most aggressive and widespread of the plants featured in this section. I have seen entire hillsides of it growing at local parks. It grows to enormous heights of 10 feet or more, and the stems can be 2 inches in diameter! It can be mistaken for plants like wild carrot with catastrophic results. This plant has no relation to western hemlock (*Tsuga heterophylla*). Avoid harvesting near this plant, as it is a common victim of chemical herbicides.

Poison hemlock is a central nervous system blocker that causes paralysis that begins at the feet and moves upward until it reaches the lungs and causes asphyxiation.

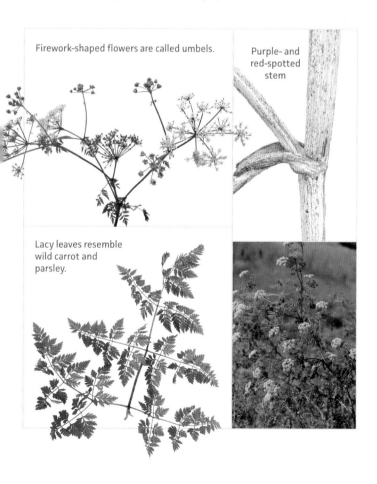

Firework-shaped flowers are called umbels.

Purple- and red-spotted stem

Lacy leaves resemble wild carrot and parsley.

Acknowledgments

This book would not have been possible without my Kickstarter community: 407 people chose to support this project financially, which allowed me to put in the number of hours needed to create the guide I envisioned.

Initially, I chose to self-publish this guide, and producing every aspect of it was a life-defining challenge for me. Normally I am a do-everything-myself kind of woman, but the monumental task of creating and self-publishing this book taught me the power of asking for help. Out of all the things this book has given me, that is the most valuable. More is possible when we work together.

After letting that lesson soak in, I quickly realized that self-publishing was going to take time away from me being out in the field doing what I love. That's when I sought out Mountaineers Books to take this precious book under their wing. It was a joy to watch the book get polished by their professional and capable hands into what you are holding right now. Thanks to all the folks at Mountaineers Books!

I want to thank my talented initial editor, Isabelle Heyward, who spent countless hours helping me make each section as clear as possible. I also want to thank my initial copyeditor, Corinne Mooney, who meticulously scoured these pages for errors. Once I brought Mountaineers Books on to this project, Erin Cusick and Janet Kimball undertook a second editing process in which they used their magic and close attention to get things even more clear and concise. Thanks so much to both of them!

Thank you to Danny Najera, who went out in the field with me several times, helped with photography, gave me crucial moral support, and inspired me constantly.

My friend Megan Acosta listened to me talk through every single stage of this project.

My mom spent countless hours reading, editing, and gently convincing me to see things a different way. She challenged me throughout the whole process to take all the steps needed.

The photography for this book was a monumental task. My friend and professional photographer Wren Morrow went out in the field with me several times to capture some of the most striking images in this book. I am grateful to Craig Althen and Ben Legler, who gave me permission to use their photographs from the Burke Museum Herbarium at the University of Washington. Their photos helped fill the gaps that appeared during the design process. Several other people also helped me take pictures in the field, including Firelight Hammerquist, Kristin Montgomery, my mom, and my dad. And finally, thank you to V. Babida and Julien Bacon for their photos.

Thanks to Kate Sinon, who helped me with the tincture ratios and alcohol-percentage recommendations and also went out in the field with me several times, along with Diana Law.

I'm grateful for those who generously contributed their recipes: Cricket McCormick, Elise Krohn, Diana Law, and Suzanne Talbert.

I want to give a special shout-out to a dedicated community of alums from my school: Audrey, Becky, Christine, Daniela, Donna, Duffy, Kristin M., Kristin R., Mardi, Vee, Zo, and others.

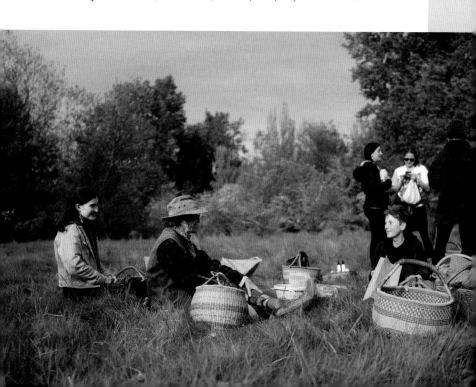

They appear in many photos in this book and made many of the field trips required for this book extremely fun.

Thanks to these special donors from my Kickstarter community whose extra donations made this book possible:

4 Sisters Holistic Remedies
AnaMichelle
Betsy Bertiaux
Jade Block
Tom Booster and Cynthia Hartwig
Nolan Bradley
Stephen T. Brown
Thomas Brown
Anna Constant
Paula Dalrymple
Danny (GRC)
David and Molly
Megan Davies and Giovanni Acosta
Eve Dixon
Sharon Duncan
Duvall Herb Farm
Hécbel C. Igartúa García
Jesse Gipe
Christine Glynn
Kenji C. Green
Jerry and Sally Gregg
Vincent Grotkopp
Megan Gurule of Wild Women Herbs
Fred and Sydney Hammerquist
Irelie and Hollyn Hammerquist
Denise Harris
Jennifer and Dale Hartley
Rebecca Hartness
The Herbal Wise Guy
Joanna Hobson
Chia Bao Hui
Hull Family
Benita Jangala
Jeff Jones
Leanne Posick Kaukola
Kim
Chris Koss
Ken and Mary Krass

Mardi Ledbetter and the 2021 Rabbit Holers
Jonny Locher
Bobbi Long
Maryn
Breanne Naparan
Joyce Netishen
The Nickerson Family: Kelly Ann, Chris, Elsie, and Elliot
Gerry Olson and Lea Johnson
Pedro
Howard Phillips
PoeM
Sara Poore
Tom Posey
Donna Ramos
Leia Ray
Jesús Segura
Sharmon and Peter
Tiffany Shuck
Sonja Sivesind
Erica Skinner
Deena D. Stevens
Tairyn Tennyson
Jennifer "J. T." Thames
Hannah van Seeters
Sarah Warner
Carol Weisbecker and Mike Ernst Leigh Brewer
Tracy Wise
Matt Wurdeman
Michelle Yang

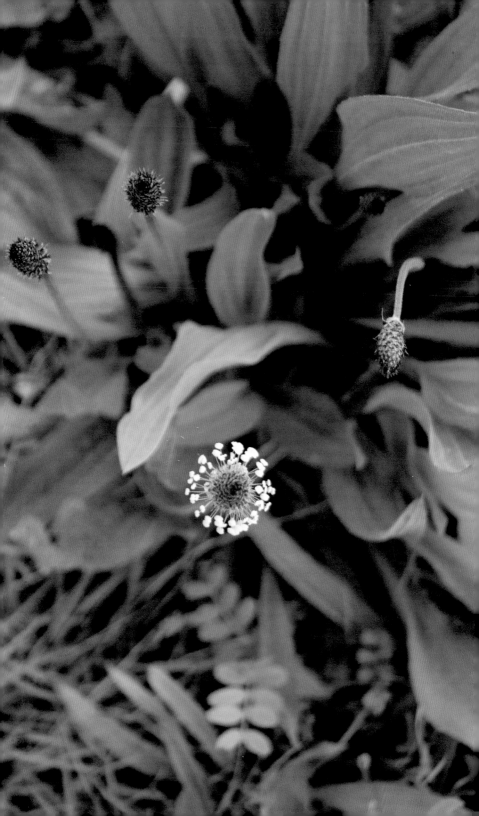

Resources

I highly encourage you to do further research and to dig into some of the following resources to learn more. Plant ID is a life-long endeavor, and I have used many of the following resources in my own learning journey and in the creation of this book. I have also included some places to purchase medicine-making supplies, dried herbs, and tinctures.

Herbalism

Books

Gladstar, Rosemary. *Rosemary Gladstar's Medicinal Herbs: A Beginner's Guide.* North Adams, MA: Storey, 2012. Covers the fundamentals, including basic cultivated herbs and recipes.

Groves, Maria Nöel. *Body into Balance: An Herbal Guide to Holistic Self-Care.* North Adams, MA: Storey, 2016. A fantastic deep dive into herbalism exploring how to use herbs and how the body works.

Hoffman, David. *Medical Herbalism: The Science and Practice of Herbal Medicine.* New York: Healing Arts Press, 2003. Focuses on specific illnesses and includes recipes.

Mars, Brigitte. *The Desktop Guide to Herbal Medicine.* 2nd ed. Laguna Beach, CA: Basic Health, 2014. A great resource about the uses of herbs.

Online

Chestnut School of Herbal Medicine
https://chestnutherbs.com
A popular online school that also has an extensive blog that I love.

HerbRally
www.herbrally.com
A subscription learning service that also has some free content.

Learning Herbs
https://learningherbs.com/free-herbal-remedies
A blog and also a subscription-based learning platform.

Plant ID and Plant Families

The Biota of North America Program (website)
http://bonap.org
This website has a distribution map that is extremely helpful to see where things grow, along with some other interesting resources.

Botany in a Day: The Patterns Method of Plant Identification, 6th Ed. by Thomas J. Elpel (book)
(Pony, MT: HOPS Press, 2013) A great place to start looking at plant families.

Burke Herbarium Image Collection (website)
https://burkeherbarium.org/imagecollection
Pictures, maps, and descriptions of all the naturalized plant species in Washington. This is one of the resources that I rely on most heavily in my work.

Calflora (website)
www.calflora.org
Lists all the naturalized plants of California.

Flora of Eastern Washington and Adjacent Idaho (website)
https://inside.ewu.edu/ewflora/
Not as detailed and extensive as other sites, but does focus on the drier parts of the region, which is valuable.

iNaturalist (website)
www.inaturalist.org
A citizen science website where folks can upload pictures of organisms (plants, animals, fungi, insects, etc.) and enter information. Go to their site and enter the scientific name of a plant and explore from there!

OregonFlora (website)
https://oregonflora.org
Naturalized plants of Oregon.

Oregon Flora Image Project (website)
www.botany.hawaii.edu/faculty/carr/ofp/ofp_index.htm
Especially great for photos of plants.

Resources for Medicine Making

Herb Pharm
www.herb-pharm.com
High-quality herbal tinctures. Based in Oregon.

Mountain Rose Herbs
https://mountainroseherbs.com
Organic dried herbs, medicine-making equipment, materials, and teas.
Based in Oregon.

Organic Alcohol Company
https://organicalcohol.com
High-quality and high-proof alcohol for making tinctures and other
projects.

Specialty Bottle
www.specialtybottle.com
Low-priced glass bottles, salve tins, and jars. Based in Seattle.

References

Culpeper, Nicholas. *Culpeper's Complete Herbal: Consisting of a Comprehensive Description of Nearly All Herbs with Their Medicinal Properties and Directions for Compounding the Medicines Extracted from Them.* London: W. Foulsham, 1975.

Grieve, Maud. *A Modern Herbal: The Medicinal, Culinary, Cosmetic and Economic Properties, Cultivation and Folk-Lore of Herbs, Grasses, Fungi, Shrubs, and Trees with All Their Modern Scientific Uses.* 2 vols. New York: Dover, 1982.

Gunther, Erna. *Ethnobotany of Western Washington: The Knowledge and Use of Indigenous Plants by Native Americans.* Seattle: University of Washington Press, 1992.

Kartesz, J. T., The Biota of North America Program. "BONAP's North American Plant Atlas (NAPA)." Last updated December 15, 2014. http://bonap.net/napa.

Kloos, Scott. *Pacific Northwest Medicinal Plants: Identify, Harvest, and Use 120 Wild Herbs for Health and Wellness.* Portland, OR: Timber Press, 2017.

McCune, Bruce, and Linda Geiser. *Macrolichens of the Pacific Northwest*, 3rd ed. Corvallis: Oregon State University Press, 2023.

University of Washington Herbarium. "Vascular Plants, Macrofungi, & Lichenized Fungi of Washington State." Accessed November 13, 2022. https://burkeherbarium.org/imagecollection/.

Recipe Index

Index

About the Author

Like many others in this field, I was drawn to herbalism because of health challenges. Herbal medicine, nutrition, and other forms of natural healing have allowed me to live a normal life, and for that I am deeply grateful. I am a relentless optimist. I believe in solutions. I believe we have great power to shift our health.

The very first herbal class I took was with Michael "Skeeter" Pilarski in Olympia, Washington, in 2009. I had discovered herbal medicine a year earlier, and I was thirsty for knowledge. The class was on wildcrafting medicinal plants in the Pacific Northwest, and I remember taking pages and pages of extensive notes. After that class, I ventured out into the woods and started harvesting wild plants, which have been my most consistent teacher throughout my career.

I studied for two years with Cascade Anderson Geller, who had a profound impact on my approach to the human side of herbalism. I sought out

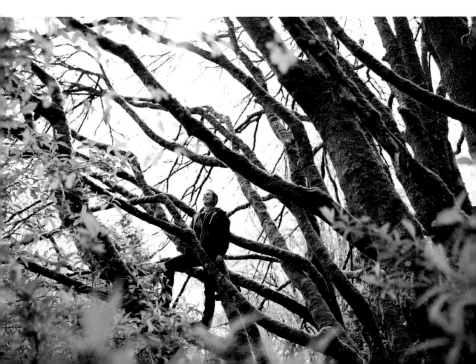

conferences, weekend intensives, and any opportunity to learn. I bought every book I could find. I harvested things, made all kinds of concoctions, experimented on myself, ate wild foods, and spent countless hours out in the field.

The most instrumental class I have taken so far was Field Plant Taxonomy with Frederica Bowcutt at the Evergreen State College, my alma mater. That class not only provided me with a deep understanding of plant morphology and how plants are related, but also instilled a love of being out in the field and of observing deeply. Our focus in the class was on the unique ecosystems and cultural history of the South Puget Sound prairies. As a class, we participated in writing and illustrating a field guide—published as *Vascular Plants of the South Sound Prairies*—which I was part of designing. That project set me up with the skills to create this book.

In 2016, I founded the Adiantum School of Plant Medicine and began leading plant walks and teaching comprehensive programs, medicine-making classes, basket weaving, and anything I am passionate about at the moment. I teach mostly outdoors, where my students and I can touch, taste, feel, listen, and look.

Visit adiantumschool.com for more information about my school.

About Skipstone

Skipstone is an imprint of independent, nonprofit publisher Mountaineers Books. It features thematically related titles that promote a deeper connection to our natural world through sustainable practice and backyard activism. Our readers live smart, play well, and typically engage with the community around them. Skipstone guides explore healthy lifestyles and how an outdoor life relates to the well-being of our planet, as well as of our own neighborhoods. Sustainable foods and gardens; healthful living; realistic and doable conservation at home; modern aspirations for community—Skipstone tries to address such topics in ways that emphasize active living, local and grassroots practices, and a small footprint.

Our hope is that Skipstone books will inspire you to effect change without losing your sense of humor, to celebrate the freedom and generosity of a life outdoors, and to move forward with gentle leaps or breathtaking bounds.

All of our publications, as part of our 501(c)(3) nonprofit program, are made possible through the generosity of donors and through sales of 700 titles on outdoor recreation, sustainable lifestyle, and conservation. To donate, purchase books, or learn more, visit us online:

www.skipstonebooks.org | www.mountaineersbooks.org

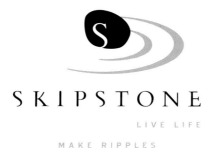

SKIPSTONE

LIVE LIFE

MAKE RIPPLES

OTHER TITLES YOU MIGHT ENJOY FROM MOUNTAINEERS BOOKS

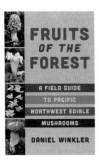

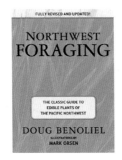

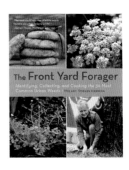

**Fruits of the Forest:
A Field Guide to Pacific
Northwest Edible
Mushrooms**
Daniel Winkler
Discover how to find,
identify, and prepare
mushrooms from Northern
California to Alaska.

**Northwest Foraging:
The Classic Guide to
Edible Plants of the
Pacific Northwest**
Doug Benoliel
The standard field guide for
the region's wild foods

**The Front Yard Forager:
Identifying, Collecting, and
Cooking the 30 Most
Common Urban Weeds**
Melany Vorass Herrera
A fun, detailed field guide to
foraging in your neighborhood—
with 60 recipes

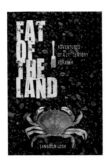

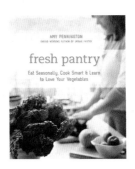

**Fat of the Land:
Adventures of a 21st
Century Forager**
Langdon Cook
A lively mix of Pacific
Northwest foraging,
natural history, food, and
outdoor adventure

**Fresh Pantry: Eat Seasonally,
Cook Smart & Learn to
Love Your Vegetables**
Amy Pennington
"Full of clever recipes for using
your kitchen to the max"
—Gwyneth Paltrow, Goop.com